NATURAL SKIN CARE AT HOME

ALSO BY LIZ MCQUERRY

Natural Soap at Home

NATURAL SKIN CARE AT HOME

How to Make Organic Moisturizers, Masks, Balms, Buffs, Scrubs, and Much More

Liz McQuerry

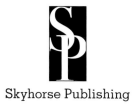

Skyhorse Publishing

Skyhorse Publishing books may be purchased in bulk at special discounts for sales promotion, corporate gifts, fund-raising, or educational purposes. Special editions can also be created to specifications. For details, contact the Special Sales Department, Skyhorse Publishing, 307 West 36th Street, 11th Floor, New York, NY 10018 or info@skyhorsepublishing.com.

Skyhorse® and Skyhorse Publishing® are registered trademarks of Skyhorse Publishing, Inc.®, a Delaware corporation.

Visit our website at www.skyhorsepublishing.com.

10 9 8 7 6 5 4 3

Library of Congress Cataloging-in-Publication Data is available on file.

Cover design by Laura Klynstra
Cover photo credit: Liz McQuerry

Print ISBN: 978-1-5107-4469-1
Ebook ISBN: 978-1-5107-4470-7

Printed in China

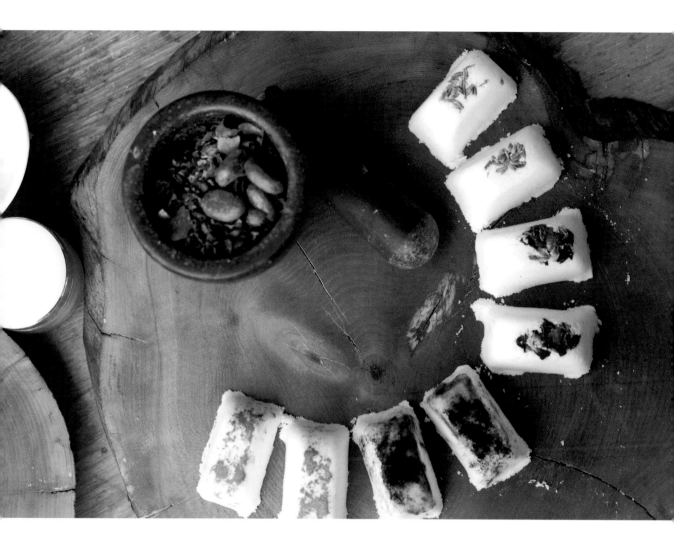

This book is devoted to you, dear reader. These are all my top-secret recipes.
May they bring you great pleasure in creating, using, and sharing.
Thank you for your support—I adore you.

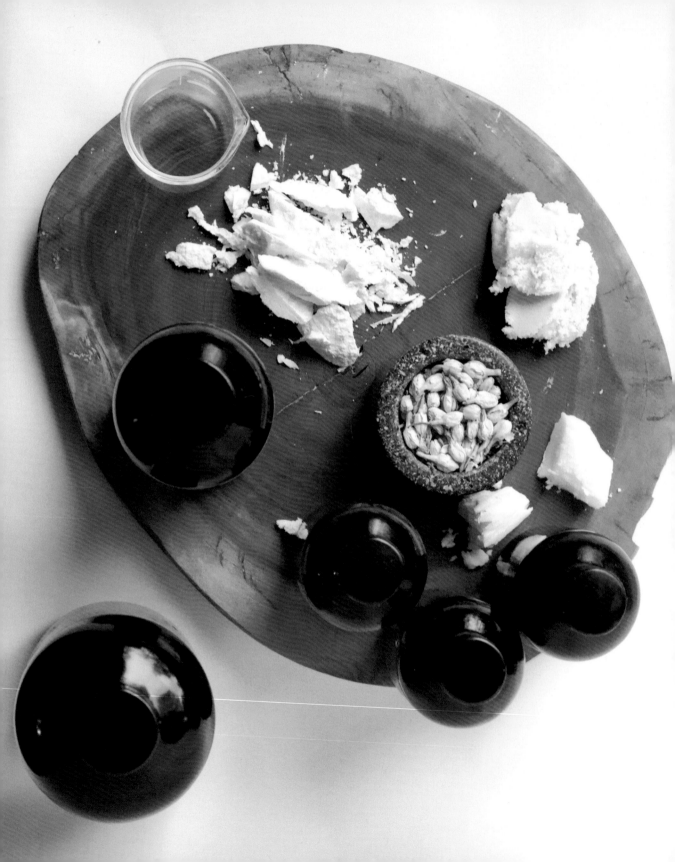

Contents

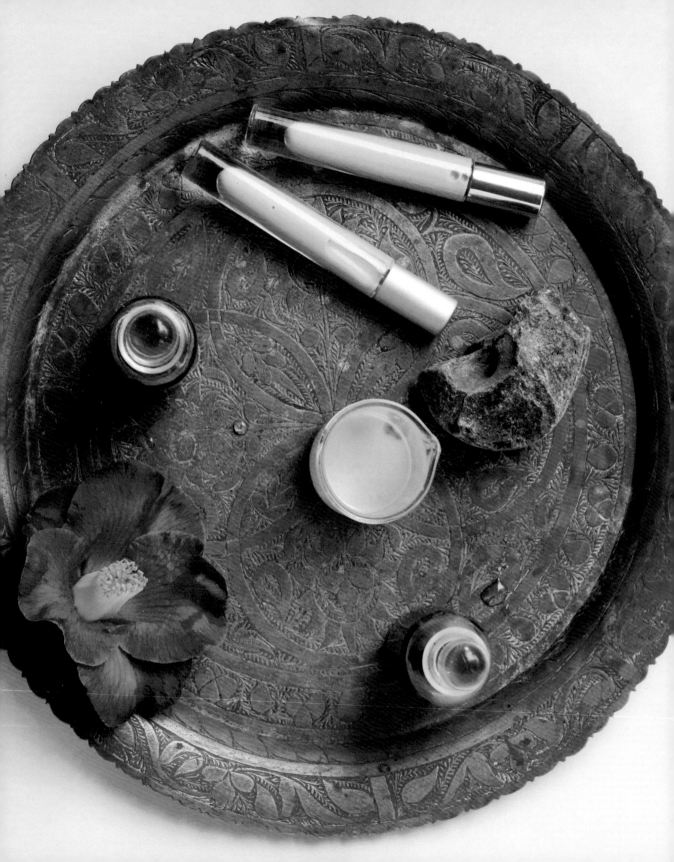

Your Introduction to At-Home Skin Care

Take your skin care into your own hands! With this book, you'll learn basic recipes and easy-to-follow prompts with clearly laid out ingredients to formulate the recipes for your own skin needs.

Skin care has come a long way from the days of humans painting their skin with Spirits of Saturn (a.k.a. venetian ceruse, a.k.a. lead) to get the whitest skin possible, leaving the skin gray and lifeless under the white painted faces, causing hair loss, and poisoning the wearer's body and mind for the sake of beauty.

While this book won't touch upon makeup, it will be covering a wide variety of ingredients you could be using to create the best skin formulations of your life!

Have you ever wondered what is in the skin care products you use? Have you examined the label and thought, *What the heck is THAT and how is it helping my skin?*

One of my favorite things about natural skin care is that it's easy to research each ingredient to learn what it does and how it will affect you. (Not to mention, most products from nature are purely good for you with zero negative side effects.)

How to Use This Book

Although this is structured like a basic recipe book, and indeed you can look up any recipe and make it just like a cookbook, this is also far more than a simple collection of recipes. This book will essentially provide you with a solid toolbelt from which you can formulate your own recipes without having a degree in science, dermatology, or cosmetology.

Each recipe is written for an average skin/hair type, but with a little perusing of the ingredients, you will quickly learn what you should plug into the recipes to make the products work for you. Many recipes include prompts that will give you clear directions to reformulate according to your skin type.

The first part introduces a variety of ingredients and is easy to reference. These ingredients have been summarized for convenience; if you choose to really get into skin care later, you'll find that the scientific information available on each is incredible, but unfortunately I can't cover all that here. (That would be an entirely different and very large book, so I leave that part up to you.)

Once we review the ingredients, you will find recipes starting with your hair and ending at your toenails—literally, head to toe. And once you've picked a few recipes to make at home that you enjoy, you can come back to check out how to package them to gift to others.

Let's get started!

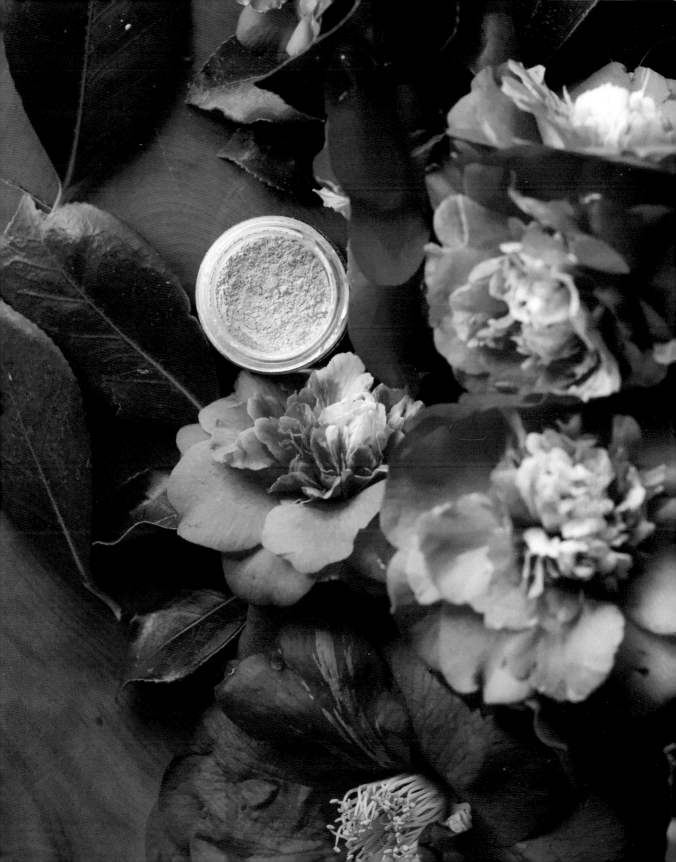

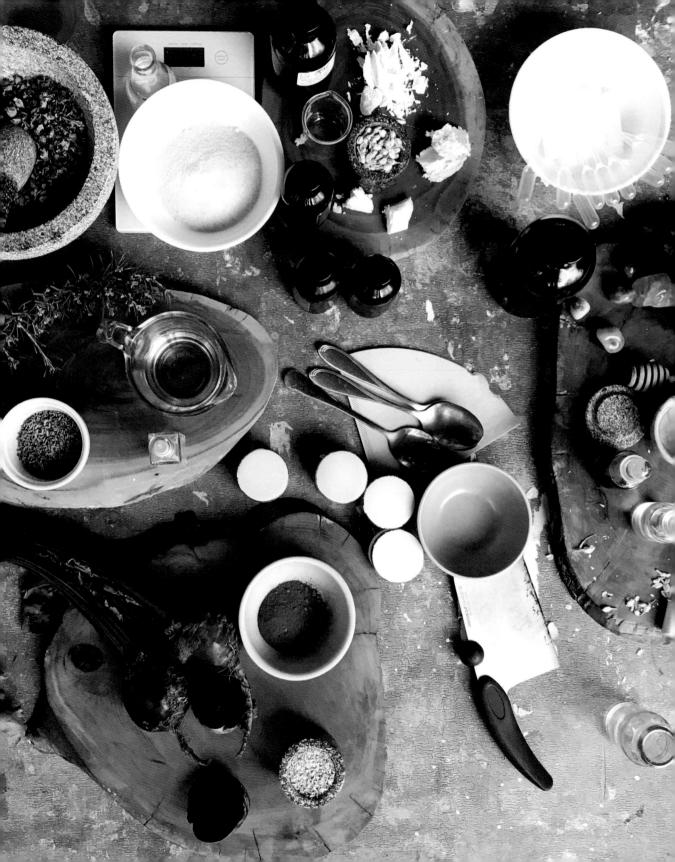

Ingredients

It's no secret: ingredients from nature are incredible.

I like the idea of making all skin care edible, because if you wouldn't put it inside your body, you must ask yourself: Should I even be putting this on my skin?

Oils

The oils chart on page 6, while not entirely extensive, covers the oils used in the recipes in this book, categorized by skin type with a little information and comedogenic rating. The comedogenic scale rates oils based on how likely they are to clog pores. This is important to be mindful of for people who are prone to acne and breakouts, as a likely-to-clog-pores oil is also likely to create blemishes. On the other hand, this scale can be used to choose a heavier oil that will stay on the skin extra long if you're prone to dry skin.

This scale is loose, as everyone's skin type will vary and be affected differently.

OIL SCALE

0: will not clog pores
1: low chance of clogging pores
2: mild chance of clogging pores
3: medium chance of clogging pores
4: quite likely will clog pores
5: almost guaranteed to clog pores

> **NOTE**
>
> When you're measuring oils, remember that 40 drops equals 1 gram. And 28 grams equals 1 ounce.

Based on this scale, non-comedogenic encompasses 0–2 ratings. These are seen as generally safe for use on skin types prone to acne.

While the comedogenic scale may be helpful, it's important to keep in mind the inherent actions of certain oils. You may choose to use a little of certain oils in a formulation because of their powerful skin care benefits even if the comedogenic number isn't the best fit for you.

Carrier oils such as sunflower, olive, and coconut can be used to make herbal oils; they are often used as a base in skin care formulas and to dilute more potent ingredients like essential oils and highly concentrated oils. Only the carrier oils are labeled *carrier*; all others are concentrated.

Concentrated oils have really high vitamin and mineral content. A little of these type of oils goes a long way, and many of them require dilution, while a few can be used straight on the skin.

The following chart on oils is not absolute; you may find varying information. Go with what works for your skin.

	comedogenic rating	carrier vs concentrated/ usage in formula	uses/actions	skin type
apricot kernel oil	2	carrier	quickly absorbing; non-greasy; antibacterial; reduces wrinkles and signs of aging; reduces redness and inflammation	dry, combination skin
argan	0	carrier	high vitamin E content; reduces acne; balances sebum production for less oily or dry skin and fewer future break outs; can also reduce scars	all skin types
black cumin seed oil	2	while this may be used straight on skin for acne spot-treating, it smells quite spicy so dilution is recommended	astringent used for acne, dry flakey skin, and irritations; anti-aging; antihistamine; firms and strengthens skin; speeds healings; scar reducing	combination to all skin types.
black raspberry seed	1-2	can be used straight on skin	maintains plumpness of skin; reduces oxidative stress	mature, acne, sensitive, and dry skin
borage	2	can be used straight on skin	anti-inflammatory; skin regenerator; reduces redness and acne	combination, sensitive, oily
camellia	1	can be used straight on skin	highly antibacterial; reduces inflammation; tones and tightens; reduces fine lines and wrinkles	acne, and all skin types
carrot seed oil	3-4	dilute	cell regenerative; heals scar tissue, age spot, wounds; stimulates poor circulation; works to heal broken capillaries; removes brown spots; reduces wrinkles	mature, dry

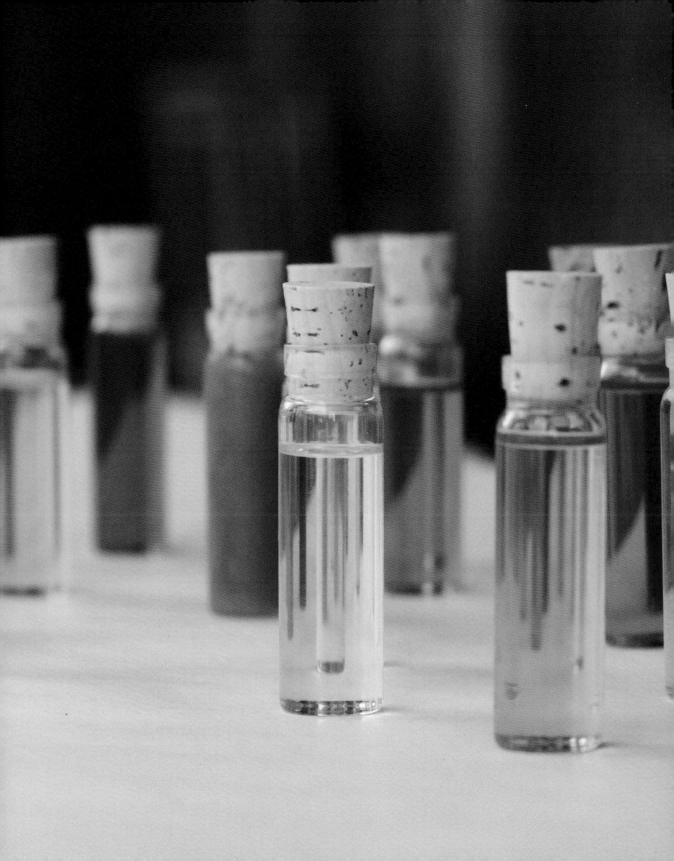

castor	1	always use diluted	a very drying oil, but feels heavy and dissipates slowly; it's the only oil with ricinoleic acid in it. It moves stagnancy throughout the body thus works well for cysts and growths; dries up acne; speeds up cell turnover	acne, oily
coconut	4	carrier	heavy oil	dry skin
evening primrose	2–3	can be used straight on skin	anti-inflammatory; enhances skin elasticity	oily, acne
grapeseed oil	1	carrier	Quickly-absorbing; non-greasy; highly moisturizing; anti-inflammatory	all skin types
hazelnut	1	carrier	antibacterial; astringent in that it reduces pore size	all, especially for acne and sensitive
hemp	0	can be used straight on skin	reduces redness and irritations; softens	all skin types
jojoba	2	can be used straight on skin and also is a carrier	imitates the skin's sebum, so it is a very good oil to use for balancing oil production	oily, but also all
meadow foam seed oil	1	can be used straight on skin	antioxidant; non-greasy; quickly absorbent; breaks down blackheads	acne, oily, sensitive
olive oil	2–3	carrier	full of nourishing squalene; reduces signs of aging; anti-inflammatory	acne, dry
pomegranate	1	can be used straight on skin	feels heavy; rich formulation of antioxidants; helps regenerate cells, keeping skin young and beautiful!	all, particularly mature
pumpkin seed	2	can be used straight on skin	Highly nutritious; packed with selenium and zinc to combat acne while enhancing healing, elasticity, and firmness	all
red raspberry seed	0–1	can be used straight on skin	Regenerative and healing; high SPF	all skin types
rose hip seed	1	can be used straight on skin	antioxidant; balances and tones skin; very nourishing	oily, acne
sea buckthorn	1	always use diluted	anti-inflammatory; regenerates cells; balances skin	all, especially dry, mature

>>

squalene or Squalane (the hydrogenated form)*	0–1	can be used straight on skin	Regenerates the skin; nourishes and heals.	all, especially mature
sunflower	0–2	carrier	light; heals skin; reduces signs of aging; shrinks pore size; balances skin tone	All
sweet almond oil	2	carrier	Helps retain moisture; enhances collagen production	dry, acne, sensitive skin types
tamanu	2	recommended to dilute (it's potent and bright yellow to green/brown in color)	thick; fragrant (kind of salty and nutty); heals scars, reduces fine lines and wrinkles	all skin types, mostly sensitive and scarred

*Squalene/Squalane: Our skin naturally produces this, but over time we produce less and our skin loses its plumpness and elasticity. Be certain if you use this that it is plant derived, as it's also found and harvested from shark liver.

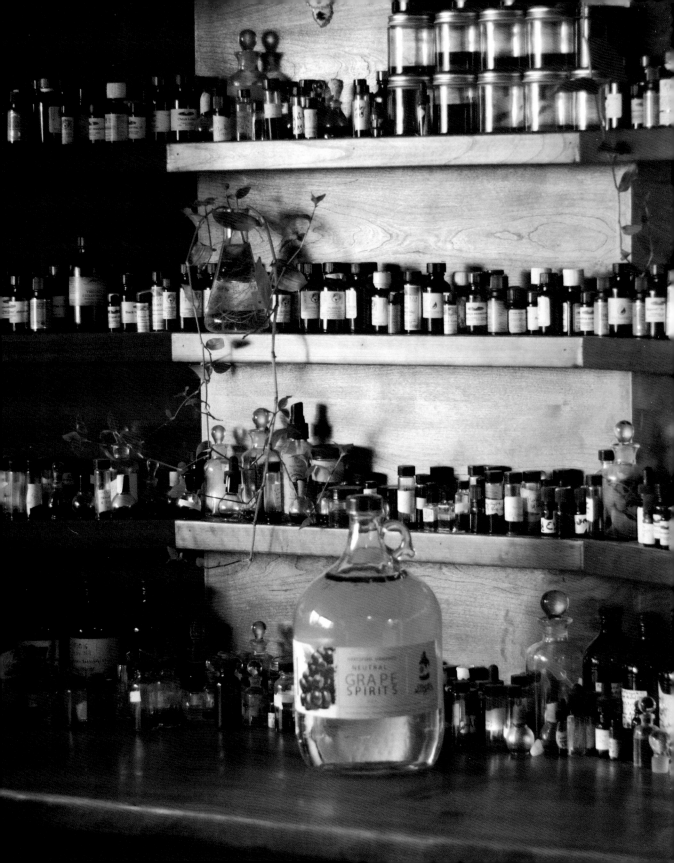

Essential Oils

A note on essential oils: always dilute these. Straight essential oil is very difficult for your system to process.

When I was in massage school, an aromatherapist lectured one night who said that when she first started mixing essential oils, they made direct contact with her skin frequently and she thought nothing of it . . . until she started getting sick. Turns out, she was overstressing her liver with the concentrated oils.

Essential oils have incredible benefits when used diluted in a carrier, so don't be afraid to use them. Just be careful.

TYPES OF ESSENTIAL OILS AND THEIR BENEFITS

Bergamot: cheery, uplifting. This oil causes photosensitivity, but it is also available as bergapten-free, meaning it doesn't contain the photosensitivity chemical.

Cardamom: spicy; stimulating; enhances circulation; warming.

Chamomile: calming; soothing; good for sensitive skin.

Cinnamon: spicy; stimulating, works to increase circulation and warm areas, enhancing blood flow. *Do not apply directly to the skin.*

Cypress: tones veins; reduces inflammations; stimulating; antibacterial.

Geranium: a sweet, rosy essential oil wonder that balances oil production for oily and combination skin types.

Frankincense: regenerative; aids in elasticity; reduces fine lines and wrinkles and even scarring

Ginger: spicy; stimulating; clearing; warming.

Ho wood: a safe alternative to the over-harvested rosewood; increases circulation; natural disinfectant; reduces inflammation.

Jasmine: skin healing; brings back a state of youthful skin.

Jasmine is my personal favorite to put immediately on burns I get while cooking. As long as I apply jasmine right away, my burns go away within a day or two without blistering.

Kapur kachri: anti-microbial; reduces inflammation and pain; enhances circulation thus aiding in hair growth, shine, and strength; stimulates the scalp thus decreasing issues like dander.

Lavender: calming; soothing.

Lemon: uplifting and oil-balancing; acne reducing; balances uneven skin tone.

Lemongrass: antibacterial; anti-fungal; antimicrobial; anti-inflammatory; uplifting; anti-anxiety; reduces acne.

Just as lemon works as a disinfectant in household cleaners, it is a wonderful and safe disinfectant in skin care preparations.

Myrrh: heals wounds; stops bleeding; stimulates circulation, can help reduce fine lines and wrinkles.

Rosemary: stimulating; clearing; antiseptic; anti-fungal with youth enhancing skin properties.

Sandalwood: excellent for mature, dry, and damaged skin; tones skin; calms skin issues such as inflammation and rashes.

Tea tree: microbial, supports healthy tissue, anti-inflammatory; clears up acne and inflamed skin issues; bacteria slaying.

Turmeric: reduces acne and inflammation; antiseptic; increases healing; reduces fine lines and wrinkles; great for all skin types.

Vetiver: anti-aging; cicatrisant; repels bugs; regenerates tissues; super strong and heavy scented.

Virginia cedar: stimulating; clearing; anti-inflammatory; repels bugs; increases hair growth; works to clear up acne; antiseptic.

Ylang ylang: seriously calming; great for reversing the signs of aging; tames acne and oily skin.

Once, while working in a hospital, the fire alarm went off on my floor. My team and I quickly ran toward the room where the alarm originated, and as we approached the door, we were greeted by the stimulating aroma of tea tree oil. Inside the room lay a bald patient with a skin condition and his wife, sitting with him and applying straight tea tree oil to his shiny scalp.

That was it, no fire. Apparently, the chemical components of tea tree are so potent that they can affect smoke detectors. Never underestimate the power of essential oils.

Herbs

Types of herbs and their benefits

Alfalfa: incredibly nourishing for the hair; builds strength, elasticity, and density.

Arrowroot: toxin drawing; skin softening with its moisture-drawing abilities; pH balancing, promotes wound healing.

Beets: full of antioxidants and skin-rejuvenating vitamins that help reverse the signs of aging and promote cellular repair.

Bhringaraj: known as the "hair herb," this beauty increases circulation to the hair follicles, creating healthy growth conditions for hair; full of nutrients that increase shine and strength; great for skin and nails; cooling.

Butcher's broom: tones veins; works on circulatory issues; helps support venous tenacity.

Chaga: adaptogen; supports cellular regeneration, healthy skin, and hair growth; full of nutrients, enzymes, and minerals.

Cocoa: full of antioxidants; aids the circulatory system; invigorates healthy skin growth.

Cordyceps: adaptogen; anti-inflammatory, system-supportive, and nourishing for healthy skin maintenance and repair; may help reduce unwanted skin growths.

Hibiscus: anti-inflammatory; clears up acne; reduces fine lines; aids in healthy cellular turnover and increased collagen productions as it is full of AHA (alpha hydroxy acids) and antioxidants; high in Vitamin C, which is great for fine lines and wrinkles.

Indigo: soothes and heals dry skin, inflammations, irritations, scaly patches; balances sebaceous glands; great for acne and oily skin.

Lavender: calming; soothing; gentle; relaxing; antibacterial; anti-inflammatory; great for treating acne.

Lemon Balm: the herb of joy; calming.

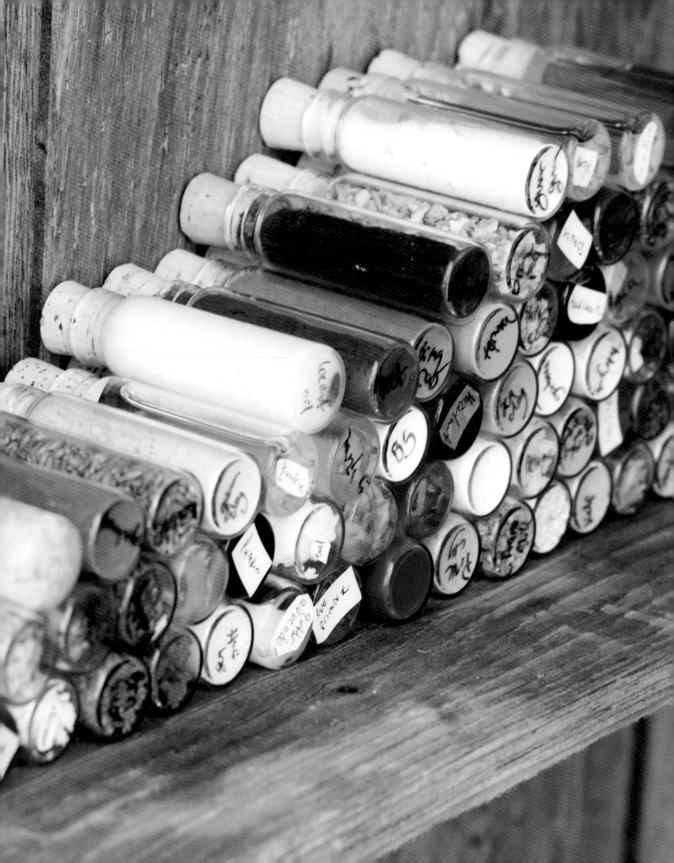

Maitake: adaptogen; full of phytochemicals to help nourish skin and heal.

Manjistha: astringent; helps support a clear complexion; calming; cooling to the skin and blemishes. Manjistha supports healthy skin by purifying the blood.

Marshmallow root: demulcent; soothing and softening; moisturizing.

Matcha: powdered green tea that draws impurities while revitalizing skin and adding nutrients.

Myrrh: reduces signs of aging; heals wounds and scars; stimulates; moves stagnation; antibacterial.

Nettle: antihistamine; full of minerals; great for skin, hair health, and healing; strength, flexibility, and nourishment for hair.

Reishi: adaptogen; supports cellular regeneration and healthy skin and hair growth; full of nutrients, enzymes, and minerals.

Roses: calms redness and irritations; cooling.

Sandalwood: gentle on skin, yet efficient; works to sooth acne and blemishes; reduces the signs of aging.

Slippery elm: moistening demulcent; hydrating.

Spirulina: a nutrient-dense algae that packs a skin-potent multivitamin with necessary enzymes for sensitive facial skin rejuvenation.

Turmeric: antiseptic, anti-inflammatory; reduces redness; reduces fine lines and wrinkles.

Clays

Types of clays and their benefits

Bentonite: contains volcanic ash and montmorillonite clay; this type of clay is very drawing and drying, thus ideal for oily skin types.

Blue: antibacterial; due to its mineral makeup, this clay is best used on oily and acne skin types.

French green: best for oily and acne skin; high in minerals.

Kaolin: the most gentle; safe for all skin; types, not very drawing, but works well for gentle absorption (like in deodorant) and exfoliation.

Pink-rose: gentle, yet efficient, this clay can be safely used on sensitive and dry skin types.

Red illite: great for oily and acne skin, highly absorbent, and can be drying (not suggested for other skin types); draws impurities from skin.

Rhassoul: best used for oily and acne skin types; rich in minerals; wonderfully toxin-drawing.

Sea: super gentle; safe for all skin types with heaps of sea nutrients.

Yellow: mellow clay, does not overly draw out oils; can be used for sensitive, dry, and all skin types.

Other Useful Ingredients

Banana flour: full of vitamins; moisturizing; oil-balancing; skin-tone balancing; makes for an excellent addition to any great skin care recipe!

Beeswax: great for all skin types and, in moderation in a formula, will not clog pores.

Charcoal: very porous and has the ability to absorb up to 500 times its surface area so it has the tendency to be very drying; an incredible cleaner that draws impurities and toxins into it amazingly well; use for oily or dry skin. *When using charcoal in products, use very sparingly.*

Chickpea powder: makes wonderful cleansing grains; exfoliates; adds proteins to skin; loaded with proteins, vitamins, minerals, and enzymes; works wonders on inflamed skin issues. You can't go wrong using this in skin care formulas.

Citric acid: a fruit- or veggie-derived acid (similar in pH to vinegar, not battery acid), used in food and skin care as a preservative. Used in bath fizzies to create a gentle chemical reaction with baking soda.

Distilled water: in natural skin care formulations, bacterial growth can occur more easily than if you are using chemicals, so be sure if you are using water in a formulation that it is distilled, so it is as clean and pure as possible.

Guar gum: can be irritating so don't use on sensitive skin types, but on the hair, it can work much like silicon, wrapping each hair in silky nutrition.

Glycerin: a humectant that supports youthful appearance of skin and allows ingredients to be better absorbed by the skin; compatible with all skin types.

Himalayan salt: high in precious minerals; balances pH; draws out impurities; definitely drying; exfoliating.

Honey: humectant; antimicrobial; antibacterial; probably the fountain of youth; keeps skin wonderfully hydrated and youthful; has the ability to clean up acne and blemishes as well as balance skin tone; works great on sunburns and irritated skin; can be applied directly to clean open wounds and speed healing while deterring bacterial growth or infection. Great for all skin types.

Hydrosols: aqueous distillates created from the liquid runoff during the process of making an essential oil; contains the aroma and nourishing attributes of the plant; awesome for facial toners!

Oats: skin softening; used in cleansing grains, as it soaks up excess oil and removes dead skin, but also good for managing acne as a moisturizing emollient; great in baths, especially if suffering from itchy, inflamed, or dry-skin issues.

Sea salt: high in precious minerals; great for the skin; pH balancing.

Sugar: exfoliant; humectant (helps skin maintain moisture); drawing; encourages new cell growth.

The following are a few natural preservatives, should you so choose to utilize these in your formulations.

PhytoCide Aspen Bark Extract: soluble in water; skin conditioning.

PhytoCide Elderberry OS: can be used in anhydrous solutions, oil solutions; skin conditioning.

Rosemary antioxidant: a natural preservative in oil formulations, derived from rosemary. Has antioxidant, skin nourishing properties.

Herbal Extractions

How to Make a Tincture

Tinctures are alcohol extractions from botanicals. You can use very little of a tincture and receive potent results because alcohol extractions are so effective. The neat thing about using tinctures in skin care is that alcohol works to absorb the substance into the skin at a rapid rate, and it's a preservative.

Note: If having alcohol in your home is an issue, make a glycerite instead. Instructions on page 22.

Use only hard alcohol when making tinctures; the higher the proof, the better. Avoid using flavored alcohols. When I started making tinctures, I would use 80-proof organic vodka because it was what I had available. Now I get my alcohol out of state and use 190-proof organic grape alcohol; it has a minimal sweet aroma, but it's hardly noticeable. I love Organic Alcohol Co!

Check out the references in the back of this book for a link to a variety of really neat alcohols.

In addition to type of alcohol used, it's also important to take the odor of alcohol into consideration in skin care tinctures as well as its color. Use what you can get your hands on, but clear is preferable if you're extracting herbs for colors.

The following will get you started with fresh herbs.

FRESH HERB TINCTURE

Fresh herbs of choice
Alcohol of choice

Fill up any size bottle to 1 inch from the top with fresh herbs, pour alcohol over herbs, cap, date, and label. Shake daily, then strain after 2 to 4 weeks. Compost your plant material, and that's it! Technically, tinctures can be kept indefinitely.

You will notice with fresh plants that not many retain their color; they will still retain their medicinal properties.

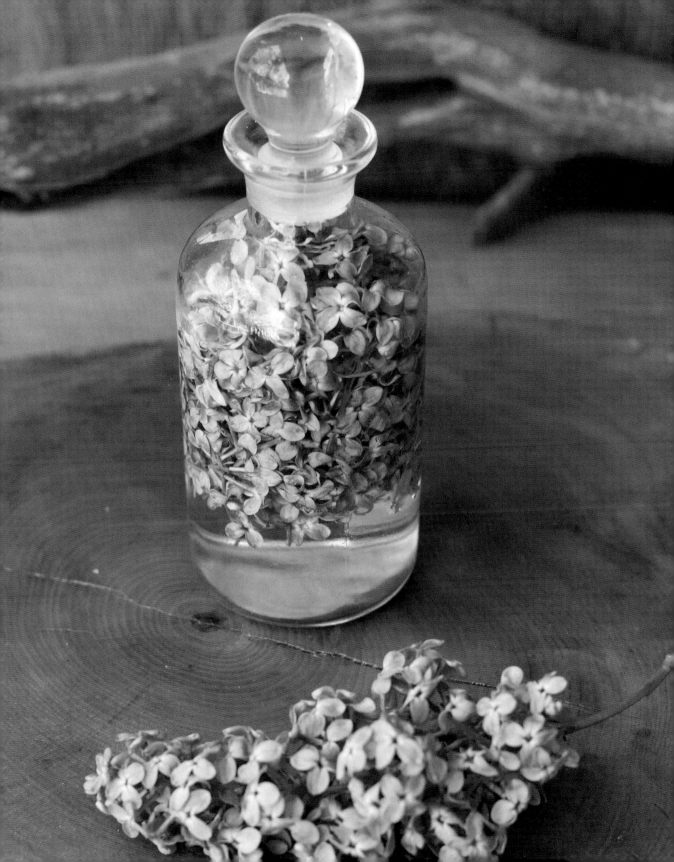

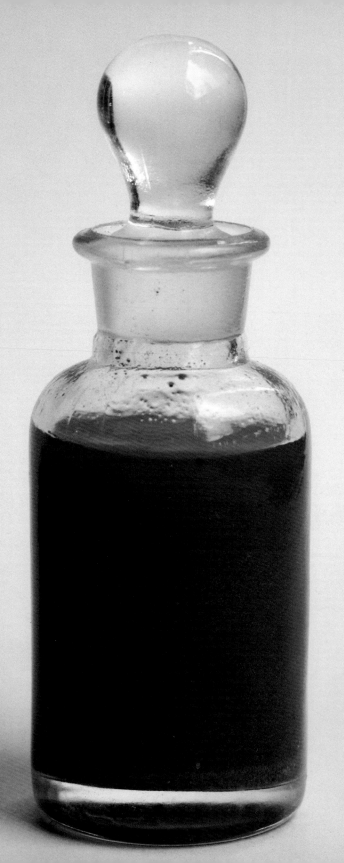

I have found with resins that I don't need to use very much to achieve great results, which is convenient and affordable! This photo is my Dragon's Blood Tincture (see page 21 for recipe).

RESIN TINCTURE BASE

2 tablespoons ground resin
8 ounces alcohol of choice

Fill your bottle with ground resin, add alcohol, date, and label. Shake daily, and strain after 2 to 4 weeks. (Personally, I only strain this type of tincture just before I use it, as resins hold up really well.)

DRIED PLANT TINCTURE

Dried plants of choice
Alcohol of choice

Similar to the Fresh Herb Tincture on page 18, fill up bottle to 1½ inches from top with plant, and add alcohol to 1 inch below the top of container. Cap, date, and label. Shake daily, then strain after 2 to 4 weeks. Compost your strained plant material.

COLOR TINCTURES

Every plant harvest will be different—sometimes the colors will be more potent, other times weaker. Sometimes things like alkanet will range from red to burgundy to purple based upon where it was grown, how the soil was, how the environment is, etc.

Here are some examples if you're looking to draw out a specific color for your skin care product:

Red to Orange

manjistha + alcohol

Purple to Red

alkanet + alcohol

Green

chlorophyll + alcohol

Yellow to Orange

turmeric + alcohol

Orange to Peach

red sandalwood + alcohol

Glycerite

Created from glycerin, these are a wonderful alternative to tinctures and can be used in hydrating skin formulas.

BASIC GLYCERITE

⅓ ounce dried herb of choice

¾ cup glycerin

¼ cup distilled water

> *I recommend using dried herb for all glycerites; fresh herbs have so much moisture they can cause a formula to turn rancid.*

Put all ingredients in a jar, cap, label, and date. Shake daily, and strain after 2 to 4 weeks. Compost plant material. This will keep for 12 to 24 months.

Oil Extractions

Oil extractions are used to extract parts of plant material. You can use any carrier oil you like for these, but it is recommended to only use dried herbs because any moisture in oil will cause it to mold quickly.

BASIC OIL EXTRACTION

⅓ ounce dried herbs

1 cup oil of choice

Put all ingredients in a jar, cap, label, and date. Shake daily, and strain after 2 to 4 weeks. Compost plant material. Oils will keep for about a year.

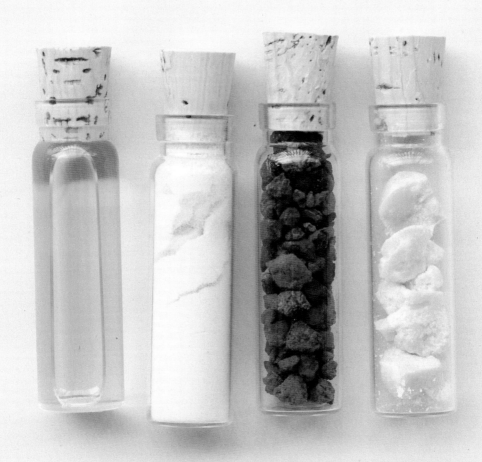

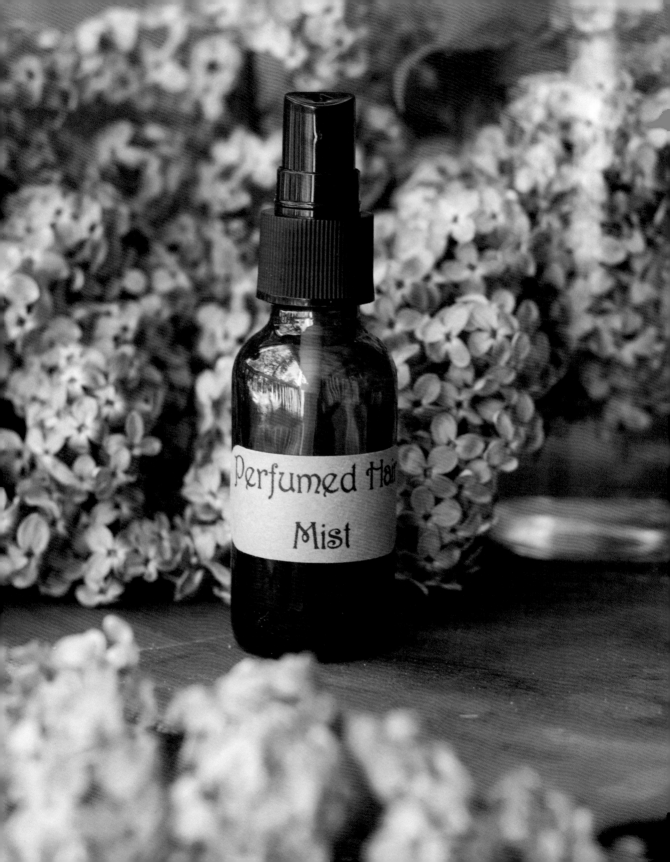

Perfumed Hair

Mist

Head-to-Toe Recipes

These recipes are organized from the top of the head down, so it is easy to focus on one area or pick and choose recipes for a hair-to-toe experience. Using natural ingredients in skin care fresh is best. These recipes all have a shelf life of around a year.

HAIR

Hair oils increase strength, improve elasticity, and moisturize your hair. And don't forget about facial hair! An often overlooked area, the beard or mustache should be given as much attention and care as any hair.

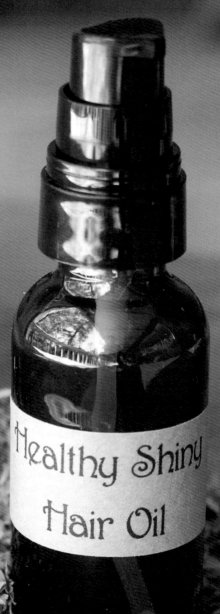

Healthy Shiny Hair Oil

Healthy hair and scalp oil, for shiny strong tresses! The following recipe is a great basic hair health recipe for daily use and frizz control without weighing down hair.

3 ounces alfalfa herbal oil in olive oil
  (for instructions to make an herbal oil go to page 22)
½ ounce almond oil
½ ounces sunflower oil
3 drops ylang ylang essential oil
5 drops kapur kachri essential oil
7 drops lemon essential oil
8 drops lavender essential oil
2 drops bergamot essential oil

Makes about 5 ounces.

Add all ingredients into clean mixing container with a pourable spout and stir well with spoon. Pour into jars with a dropper for clean, easy use and then label.

To use, after showering and drying hair with a towel, place about 10 drops of this oil into your hands and rub hands together. Starting at tips of your hair, scrunch into hair, moving hands upwards. Rub into your scalp, increasing cranial circulation, and work your hands back down, mixing oil in thoroughly.

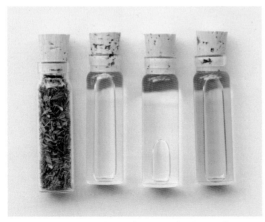

HAIR OIL PROMPT
What would your hair benefit from, and why?
  Now, reformulate this recipe for you using the same ingredient ratios.
  Substitutions for herbal oil could be: almond, sunflower, or an essential oil blend.

alfalfa, almond oil, sunflower oil, olive oil

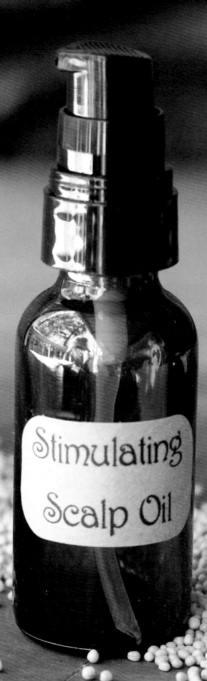

Stimulating Scalp Oil

Oftentimes, our scalp will get overly oily or incredibly dry and flaky. This blend will take care of both sides of the spectrum, balancing sebaceous glands, taming dander, and soothing itch. Use about once a week at first until your scalp gets balanced.

3 ounces mustard seed herbal oil*

1 ounce jojoba oil

1 ounce hazelnut oil

2 drops thyme essential oil

5 drops turmeric essential oil

5 drops kapur kachri essential oil

3 drops rosemary essential oil

8 drops tea tree essential oil

4 drops myrrh essential oil

* Mustard seed soaked in olive oil. See page 22 for info on herbal oil making.

Makes 5 ounces.

Mix all ingredients in a bowl, blend well, pour into bottle with a pump, and label.

To use, massage up to three pumps into scalp and let sit for half an hour. Rinse or leave until you wash your hair next.

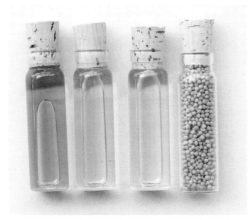

hazelnut, jojoba, sunflower, mustard seeds

NOTES

....

....

....

....

....

....

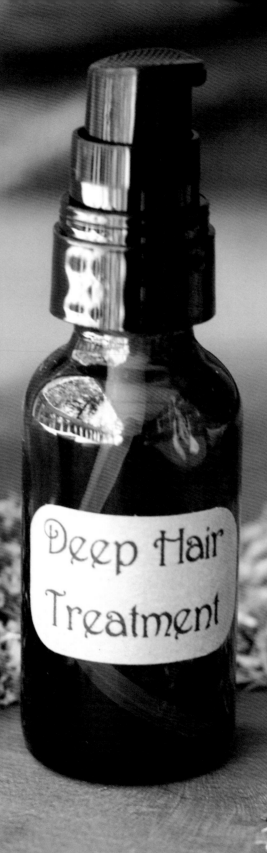

Deep Hair Treatment

This is a weekly treatment and much heavier than a basic oil. It is meant to be applied, allowed to sit, and then washed out.

I suggest using it at least once a week for hair health, especially if you have treated hair, use a blow dryer, or go in chlorinated water often. Plus, a regular serious head massage is wonderful for healthy scalp circulation and imperative in paying attention to your body from head to toe.

3 ounces horsetail herb in olive oil
  (see page 22)
2 ounces alfalfa herbal oil in olive oil
  (see page 22)
2 ounces jojoba oil
2 ounces almond oil

3 drops tea tree essential oil
3 drops kapur kachuri essential oil
3 drops lemon essential oil
3 drops lavender
3 drops frankincense

Makes 9 ounces.

Stir all ingredients until well mixed. Pour into containers with pump applicator. Label.

To use on wet or dry hair, massage a pump or two into the scalp and work out to the tips of your hair. If you have a lot of hair, you may end up using an entire bottle. Leave in hair for about half an hour and then wash out.

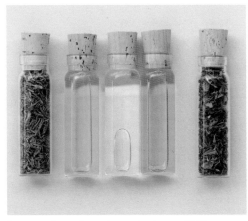

horsetail, jojoba, almond, olive, alfalfa

NOTES

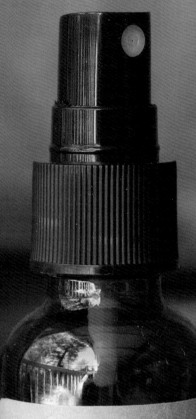

Big Hair Ocean Breeze Spritzer

Salt makes hair wild and big. Have you ever been to or even near the ocean, and noticed your hair has amassed awesome body? Well, this is ocean mist in a bottle for using any time you like!

¼ teaspoon sea salt
1 cup distilled water
essential oils of your choice, if desired

Makes 1 cup.

Mix all ingredients in a bottle with spritzer and shake until salt is dissolved. Label. Spritz over dry hair, and fluff hair with hands as it dries. Enjoy your voluptuous mane!

Perfumed Hair Mist

This super simple recipe perfumes the hair while adding the benefits of any essential oil you'd like. It's really up to you with where you want to go with it. My favorite is using a blend of Jasmine and Sandalwood essential oils. Jasmine is softening for the hair while sandalwood heals broken and damaged hair, plus it smells amazing!

1 ounce distilled water
7 drops essential oil of your choice

Makes 1 ounce.

Blend water and oil in a glass container with spritzer attachment. Shake and label. Spray onto hair as desired.

NOTES

....

....

....

....

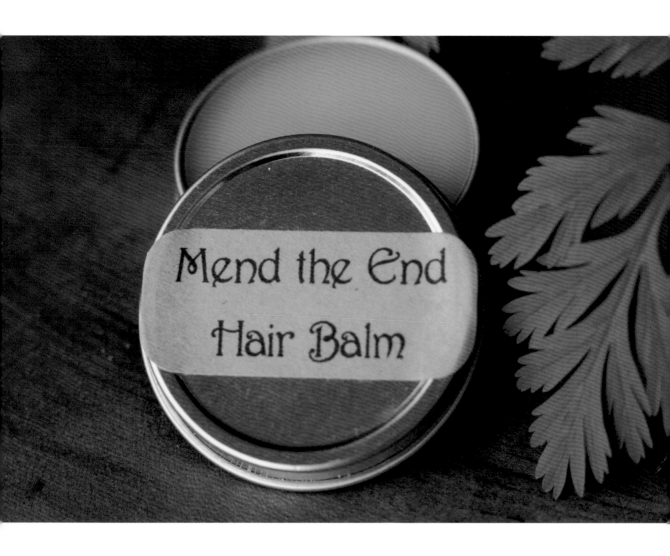

Mend the End Hair Balm

This solid hair care formulation is excellent for tip damage such as split ends, but also can be used as a hair tamer if you happen to have exceptionally frizzy hair.

72 grams coconut oil
11 grams almond oil
10 grams jojoba oil
32 grams beeswax
6 drops sea buckthorn berry oil
6 drops lavender essential oil
6 drops sandalwood essential oil

Makes about 4½ ounces.

Mix all ingredients together. Set over double boiler until melted and then pour into containers. Allow to harden, cap, and then label.

To use, massage a small amount into your hands and work into tips of hair and up to scalp.

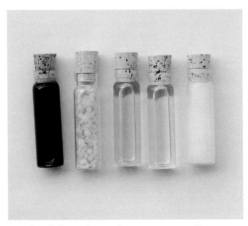

sea buckthorn berry, beeswax pastilles, jojoba, almond, coconut

NOTES

....
....
....
....
....
....
....

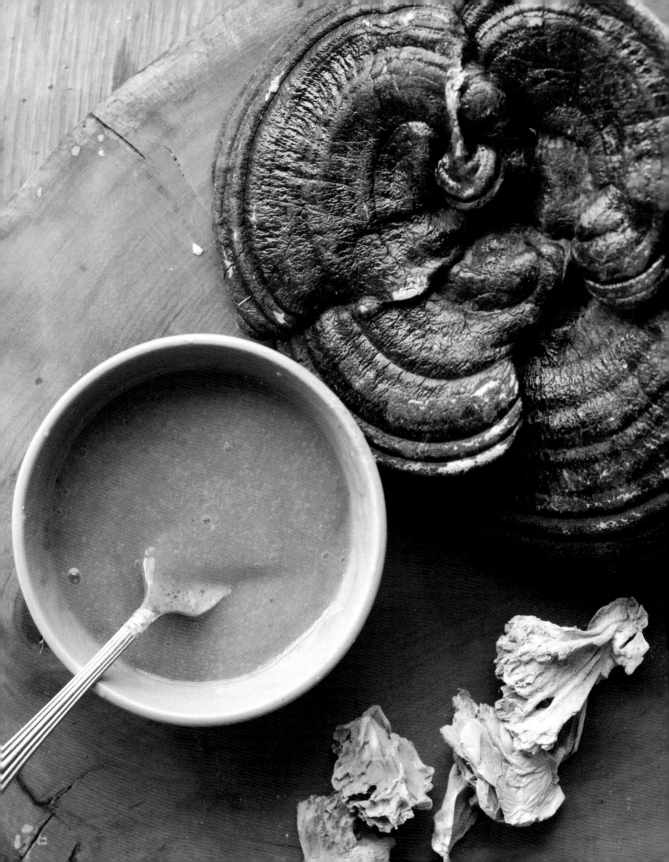

Mushroom Hair Mask

Just like a facial mask, this goes on wet and sets until dry. Then you wash it off. It serves up a powerful punch of hair vitamins and is full of adaptogenic mushrooms for healthy hair, cocoa butter to moisturize, and guar gum to help soften hair and reduce static.

1 ounce guar gum
6 grams cocoa butter, finely grated
4 grams powdered mushrooms

Makes 1½ ounces.

Mix ingredients together. Place in jars with a lid, label, and that's it!

To use, take about ½ teaspoon of powdered mix and blend in ½ cup of hot water, whipping quickly to keep guar gum from clumping. Blend well.

Apply goop to hair, massage in, let dry, and wash out. Enjoy your silky locks!

One fun thing about using guar gum in a formulation is that it will activate with any temperature of water—hot, cool, warm—however, because this recipe uses cocoa butter, you will need to mix with hot water to melt the cocoa butter.

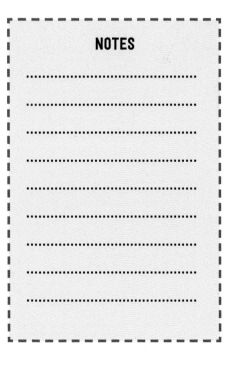

NOTES

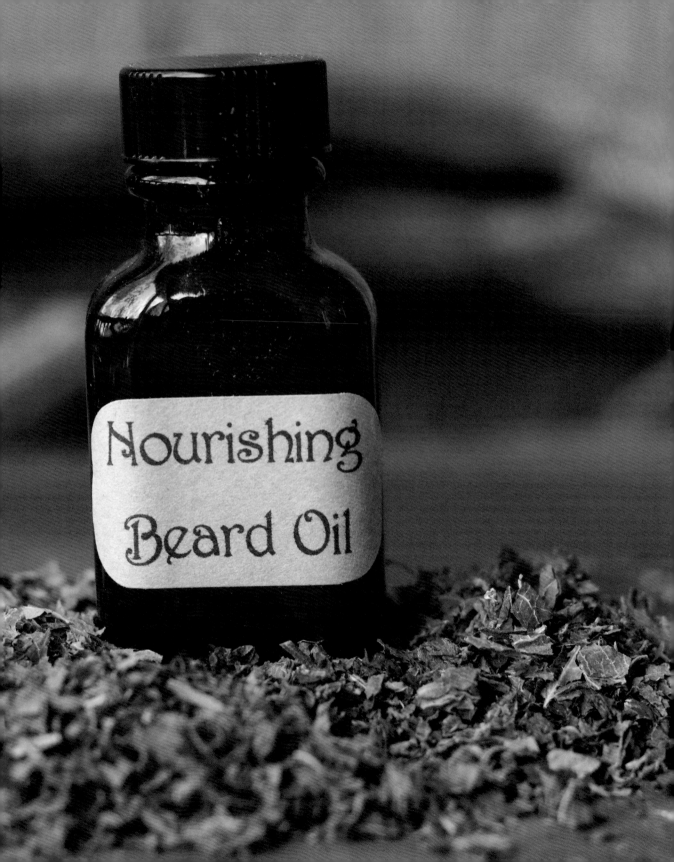

Beards!

The following recipes are created to use together for the best results. Use the hydrating beard mist, follow with beard oil, and hold your beard together with the taming conditioning beard balm.

Nourishing Beard Oil

This beard oil recipe is formulated to enhance hair elasticity and strength, stimulate growth, and soothe dryness and itching while adding serious shine without dampening the beard. This oil is applied daily for all day use, so use just a little at a time.

4 ounces nettle oil in grapeseed oil
  (see page 22)

1 ounce argan oil

1 ounce hemp oil

2 ounces apricot kernel oil

1 ounce jojoba oil

8 drops Virginia Cedar essential oil

½ drop vetiver essential oil

10 drops bergamot essential oil

3 drops lavender essential oil

Makes about 8 ounces.

Blend all ingredients together in a bowl. Pour into glass bottles with dropper tops for clean and easy application.

To use, place about three drops in your hand and rub hands together. Scrunch into beard. Next, massage beard at follicles and continue to work oil in and around until well incorporated.

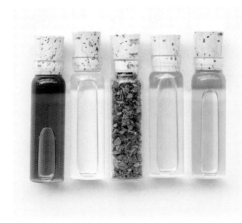

hemp, apricot, nettle, jojoba, argan

BEARD OIL PROMPT

What would your specific beard type benefit from, and why?

Now reformulate this recipe for you using the same ingredient ratios.

Substitutions may include herbal oil and other oils, if desired. Try swapping just a gram of carrier oil with one gram of rich oil, or variations on essential oil blends.

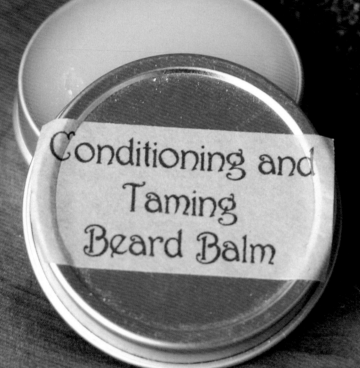
Conditioning and Taming Beard Balm

Beard Conditioning Taming Balm

This recipe has a variety of super nourishing oils specific for hair taming and health. Maintain your best beard with this conditioning balm.

1 gram pumpkin seed oil

2 grams rosehip oil

1 gram raspberry seed oil

6 drops black cumin oil

30 grams jojoba oil

8 grams beeswax

1 drop lavender essential oil

6 drops sandalwood essential oil

Makes about 1½ ounces.

Mix all ingredients together. Set over double boiler until beeswax is melted. Pour into containers and let harden, cap, and label.

To use, massage a small amount into hands and work into tips of beard and up to face. This is perfect for beard health and taming.

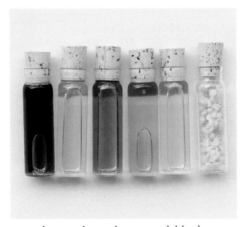

pumpkin seed, raspberry seed, black cumin, rosehip, jojoba, beeswax pastilles

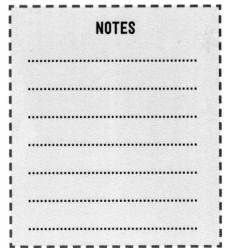

NOTES

....
....
....
....
....
....
....

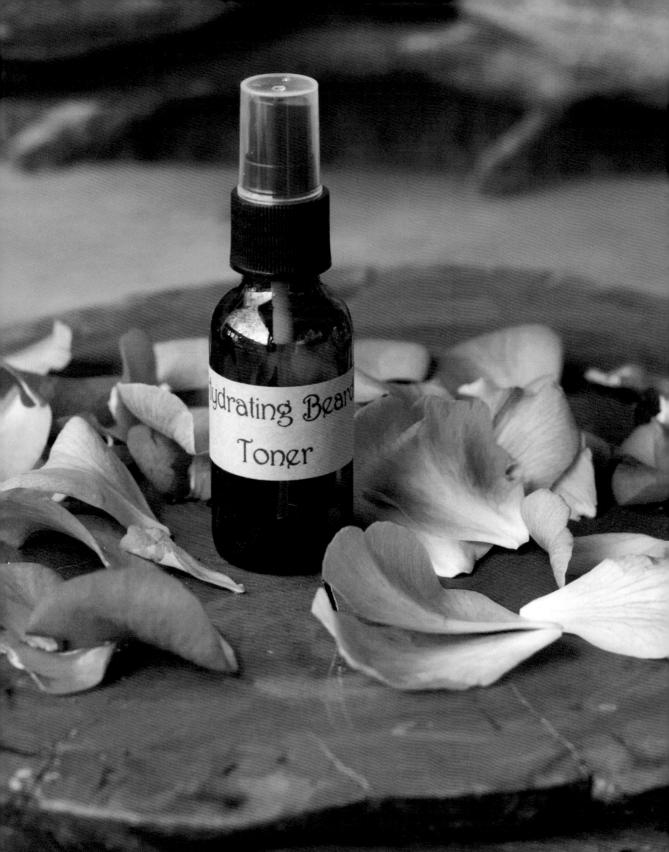

Hydrating Beard Toner

Yes, even beards can benefit from using toning hydration, especially if your beard suffers from dry, itchy patches against the skin area. This is simple yet effective and will help your beard always present attractively!

1 ounce rose hydrosol
⅛ teaspoon honey

Makes 1 ounce.

Combine in a bottle with a spray top, shake, and label. That's it!

To use, spray as needed into beard and really work it in against the skin.

This will have a short shelf life, so keep refrigerated or add a touch of natural water-based preservative.

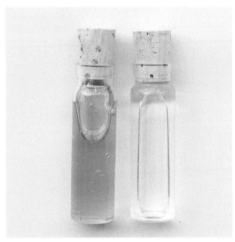

honey, rose hydrosol

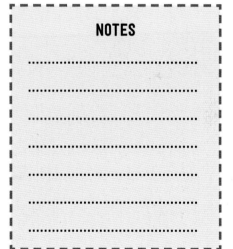

NOTES

....
....
....
....
....
....
....

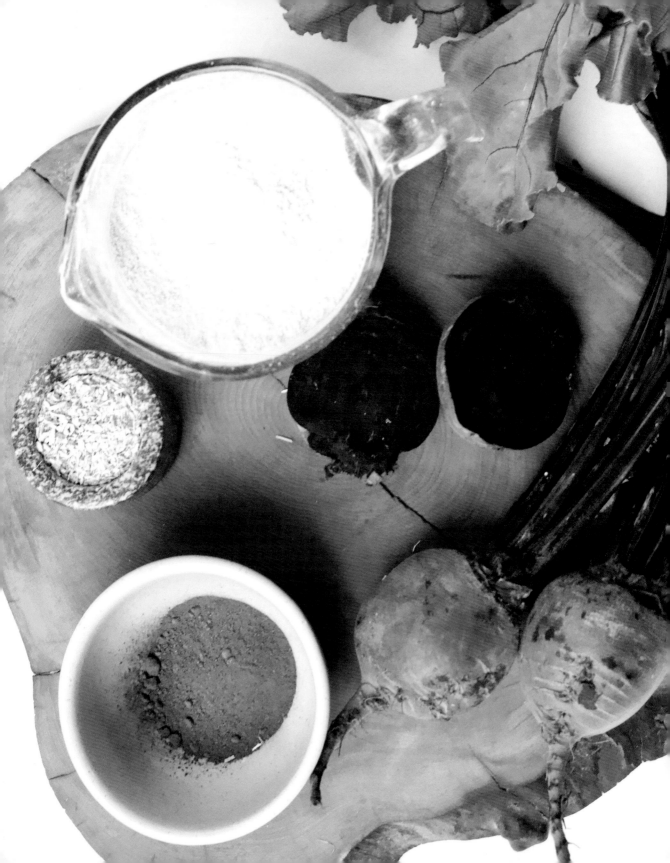

FACE

This is a great section to practice figuring out your own formulations. The following section has plenty of room and ideas for heaps of variations based on your own facial skin type. Have fun, experiment, or simply follow the recipes that sound good. The recipes start with facial cleansers and work through all-things facial, ending with moisturizers, so you can create your very own facial set by the time you're through!

Washes

Facial Cleansing Grains

The following recipe is incredibly simple, using moisturizing marshmallow root and highly nutritious beet powder. Beets are full of antioxidants and skin rejuvenating vitamins that help reverse the signs of aging and promote cellular repair.

1 cup kaolin clay
¼ cup oats, ground
3 tablespoons beet powder
1 teaspoon ground marshmallow root
3 drops immortelle essential oil
3 drops chamomile essential oil

Makes 1½ cups.

Mix all the powders and oats together. Take a tablespoon of the powder and place into a separate container. Add the essential oils to this small amount of cleansing grains and mix thoroughly. Use your hands to squish the clumps into powder. Once the scents are incorporated completely, add this small amount back to the full amount of cleansing grains and mix well. Bottle and label.

To use, wet your face, and then massage a little bit of grains into your skin. You can also choose to add some of the grains to a little water until you get a paint-like consistency and massage into face, rinse off, and follow with moisturizer.

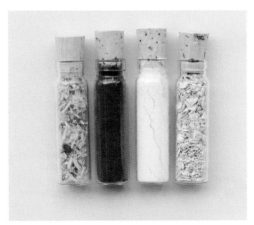

marshmallow root, powdered beet, kaolin clay, oats

FACIAL GRAINS PROMPT

Substitute your own herbs. Try adding an herbal blend. Use different grains. Get creative and don't be afraid to mix it up!

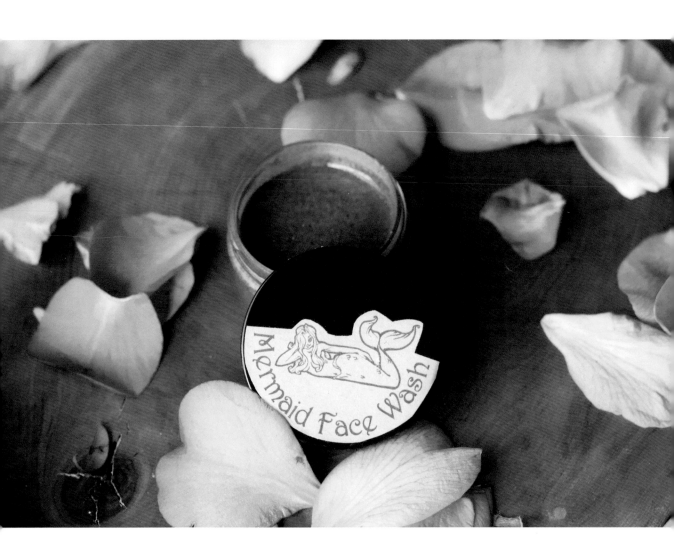

Mermaid Face Wash

This is another soap alternative that incorporates the moisturizing powers of glycerin. The formula is wonderfully astringent and nourishing but gentle.

4 ounces garbanzo flour
1 teaspoon ground lemongrass
¼ teaspoon ground kelp
½ teaspoon beet powder
6 ounces glycerin

Makes 11 ounces.

Blend all the powder ingredients together, and then slowly mix in glycerin until fully incorporated. Pour into jars, cap, and label.

To use, wet face first. Take a bit of your facial wash in your hands and scrub into face in circular motions. Rinse, then follow with toner and moisturizer if desired.

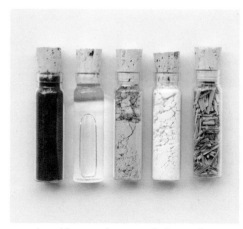

powdered beets, glycerine, kelp, garbanzo flour, lemongrass

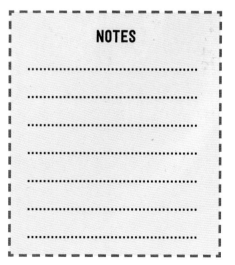

NOTES

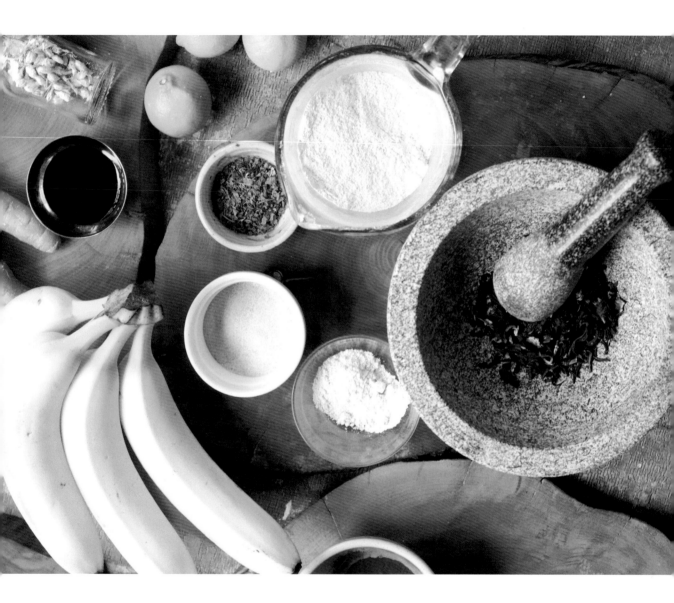

Banana Grains

This blend is very gentle and softening. Just one more recipe to share so you can see there really is no limit to facial cleanser variations.

½ cup banana flour
½ cup oat flour
¼ cup kaolin clay
¼ cup ground nettle
1 tablespoon ground hibiscus

Makes 1½ cups.

Pour all ingredients into a mixing bowl and blend well. That's it! This makes about 1½ cups of banana grains.

If you'd like to put the blend into little jars, do so now, or store in an airtight jar. Label, and enjoy!

To use, pour about a teaspoon of cleansing grains directly into your hand. If you prefer, you can add the grains to a small bowl and add enough water to get a liquid paint-like consistency. Rub into face in circular motions, wash off, and follow with toner and moisturizer. Feel the joy!

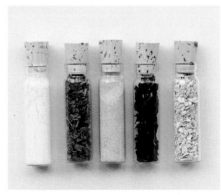

kaolin clay, nettle leaf, banana flour, hibiscus, oats

Bananas—this tropical fruit just might be your skin's new best friend. It's full of potassium, vitamin A, C, E, and more. In your body, potassium helps maintain moisture and is necessary for creating new cells. Without this hydrating nutrient, your cells die, your skin and arteries become hard, the heart has trouble moving fluids, and toxins build up. Vitamin C is necessary to produce collagen, and reduces redness, and blemishes. Vitamin E is moisturizing as well as wrinkle-, fine line-, and scar-reducing. Bananas help balance skin tone and oil production.

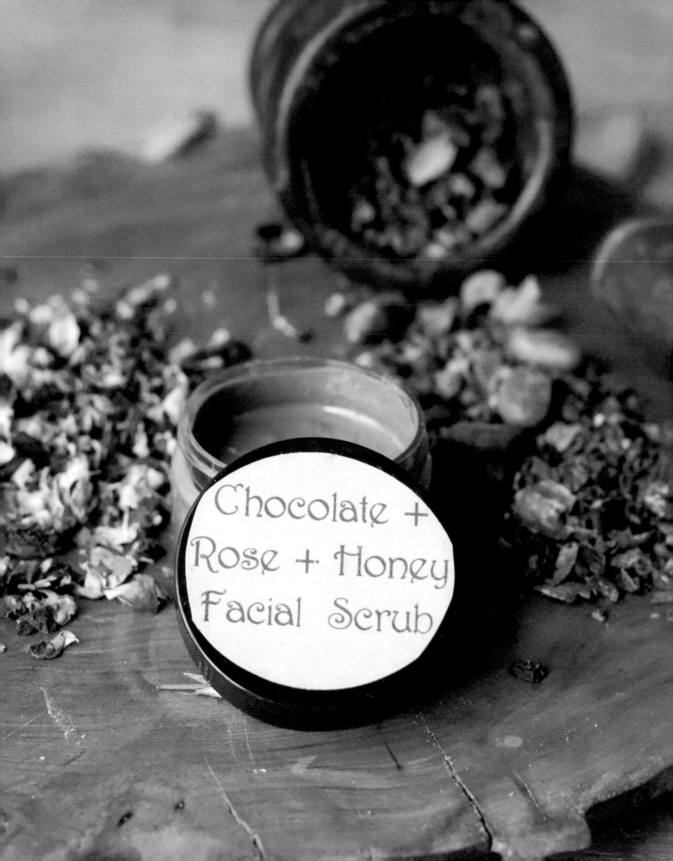

Chocolate Roses and Honey Facial Scrub

Try this smooth and creamy facial goodness for some really soft skin!

1 teaspoon ground rose petals
½ ounce cocoa powder
1 ounce kaolin clay
3 ounces honey

Makes 4½ ounces.

Stir dry ingredients together, add honey, and blend well. Honey tends to be a little tougher than glycerin to mix into formulations due to its viscosity, but it will blend in nicely eventually. Put into containers, label, and cap.

To use, wet your face, take a little bit of facial scrub into your hands, massage into face, wash off. Wowzers!

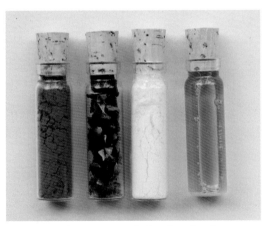

cocoa powder, rose petals, kaolin clay, honey

Chocolate is surprisingly fantastic for the skin, which really is no wonder when one considers how delicious it is. Kaolin clay is a gentle and wonderful exfoliator that shrinks pores while pulling out excess oil.

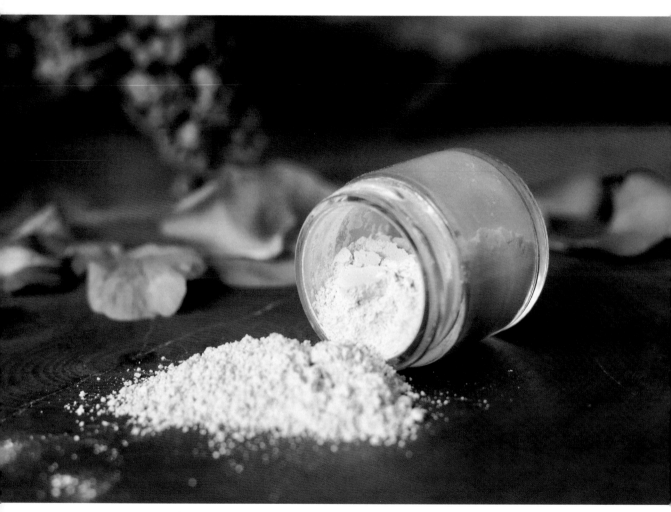

Basic Facial Mask, page 56

Masks

A NOTE ABOUT FACE MASKS

This section could fill an entire book. The idea behind a facial mask is to draw out toxins while tightening the skin. Finding the right balance of skin-tightening ingredients for your skin without leaving it flaky and dry is important. Some masks are more tightening and drying while others can be far gentler. So if you have dry, mature, or sensitive skin already, something gentle will be more suited for you than something for acne and oily skin.

The following are a wide variety of masks to get you started, but be sure to come back to the prompt when you're ready to leap off on your own formulations—I'm excited for the things you will create!

You will almost always want to follow a mask with a toner and a moisturizer, as they are very effective on the skin. This first recipe is a very basic, no-strings-attached mix; it's a good blend to start with as a base and add things to or substitute. The kaolin clay is very gentle, almost too gentle on its own, whereas bentonite is far too drying on its own, so I created this mix. It's a really nice blend, using just the right amounts of clays.

Basic Facial Mask

As I mentioned in the box on the previous page, this recipe is a very easy, no-questions-asked mix. You can use this as a base and add whatever you'd like. See the prompt below!

4 ounces kaolin clay
2 ounces bentonite clay

Makes 6 ounces.

Blend both ingredients together, pour into jars, cap, and label.

To use, place a little bit of mask in a bowl, add water until you have a paint-like consistency, massage onto face, let dry, wash off. Follow with moisturizer.

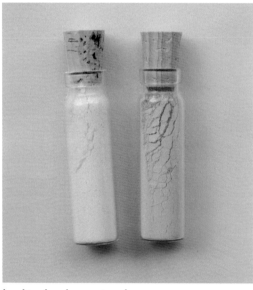

kaolin clay, bentonite clay

BASIC CLAY MASK PROMPT

As you can see, the facial mask is very easy to use for your own formulations. Go ahead and start adding your own ingredients, substituting clays, etc. I have included a number of other face mask recipes to get the idea juices flowing, but feel free to copy, tweak, or entirely reformulate any for yourself.

Jasmine Facial Mask

A deliciously aromatic skin treat, jasmine softens the skin, making a lovely balance to the drying effects of the other facial mask ingredients.

2 ounces kaolin clay

1 ounce bentonite

½ ounce powdered jasmine

3 drops jasmine sambac (or Jasmine Absolute) essential oil

Makes 3½ ounces.

Mix powdered ingredients together. Then place just about a tablespoon of powdered mixture into a mixing bowl, add essential oil, and mix with the back of a spoon. Eventually, you may need to start pinching it with your fingers to incorporate the entire tablespoon of powder. When you feel you have mixed the essential oil in as thoroughly as possible, add it back into the bigger pot of powder and mix in fully. Bottle and label.

To use, blend a little of the mask with water in a separate mixing bowl, massage into face, let dry, and wash off. Follow with moisturizer.

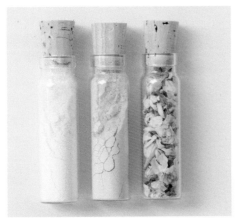

kaolin clay, bentonite clay, jasmine flowers

For an incredibly beautiful twist on the facial mask, consider incorporating essential oils for their aromatic and therapeutic qualities. This smells incredible when you apply it to skin, and the delicious scent stays after the mask is washed off. Yum!

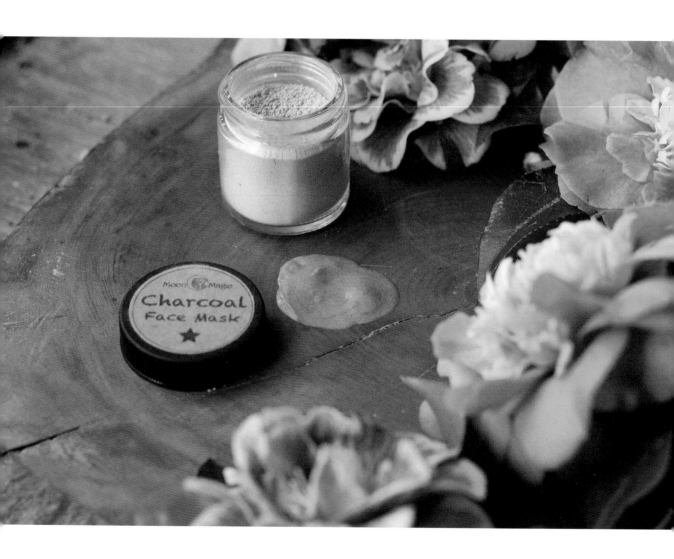

Charcoal Facial Mask

This lovely gray-hued facial mask is probably the most drying of all the facial mask recipes, making this the ideal recipe for those with oily skin.

4 ounces kaolin clay
2 ounces bentonite
1 teaspoon activated charcoal

Makes 6 ounces.

Blend ingredients together until mixed, then bottle, cap, and label.

To use, place a little bit of mask in a bowl, add water until you have a paint-like consistency, massage onto face, let dry, and wash off. Follow with moisturizer.

Keep in mind, charcoal is very absorbent thus *very* drying, so a little goes a long way.

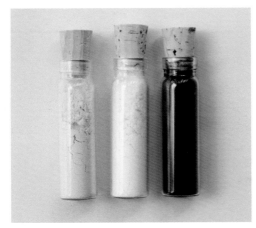

bentonite clay, kaolin clay, activated charcoal

NOTES

....
....
....
....
....
....
....

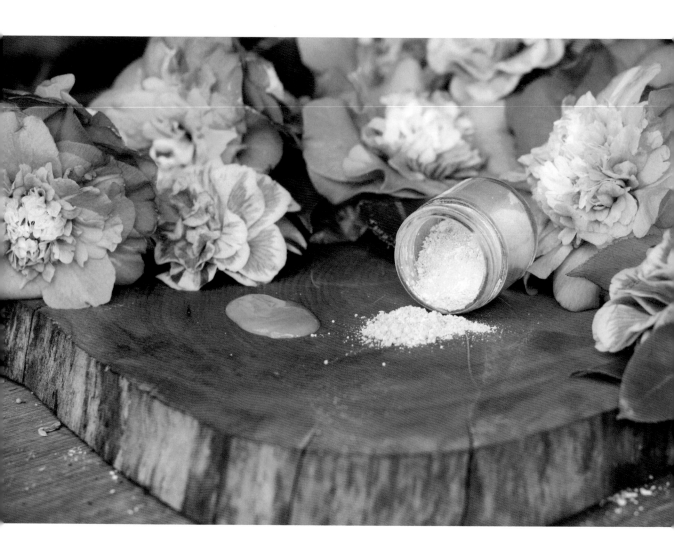

Pink Facial Mask

Pink clay is a very gentle clay. It gives this mask a fun pink hue and creates a nice facial mask for sensitive skin.

4 ounces kaolin clay
1 ounce bentonite clay
1 ounce pink clay

Makes 6 ounces.

Blend all ingredients together, pour into jars, cap, and label.

To use, place a little bit of mask in a bowl, add water until you have a paint-like consistency, massage onto face, let dry, and wash off. Follow with moisturizer.

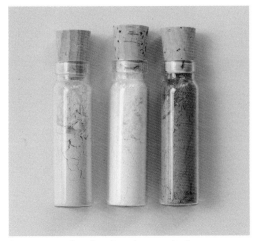

bentonite clay, kaolin clay, pink clay

NOTES

....

....

....

....

....

....

....

Indigo Facial Mask

This is a fun blue-colored facial mask. Indigo is incredible for skin health, reducing itching, dryness, and inflammation, and is found in a variety of really high end facial products.

4 ounces kaolin clay
1 ounce bentonite clay
1 ounce blue clay
1 teaspoon indigo powder

Makes 6 ounces.

Stir ingredients together until mixed, then bottle, cap, and label.

To use, place a little bit of mask in a bowl, add water until you have a paint-like consistency, massage onto face, let dry, and wash off. Follow with moisturizer.

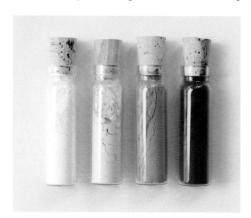

kaolin clay, bentonite, blue clay, powdered indigo

Taking our basic blend, we can add herbs and adjust clays and creat a lovely blue-hued face mask. Indigo is incredibly good for all skin types.

Siren's Blend Facial Mask

Utilize elements from the ocean for a high in skin healthy minerals facial mask.

4 ounces kaolin clay
1 ounce bentonite clay
1 ounce sea clay
1 teaspoon ground jasmine
⅛ teaspoon ground kelp

Makes 6 ounces.

Stir ingredients together until mixed, bottle, cap, and label.

To use, add a little bit of mask to a bowl, add water until you have a paint-like consistency, massage onto face, let dry, and wash off. Follow with moisturizer.

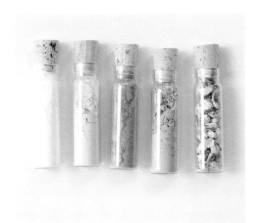

Sea clay is very gentle, jasmine is softening and soothing, and kelp is super great for the skin in counterbalancing negative effects of age and time. Rich in minerals, this blend is in my top favorites masks ever.

kaolin clay, betonite clay, sea clay, powdered kelp, jasmine flowers

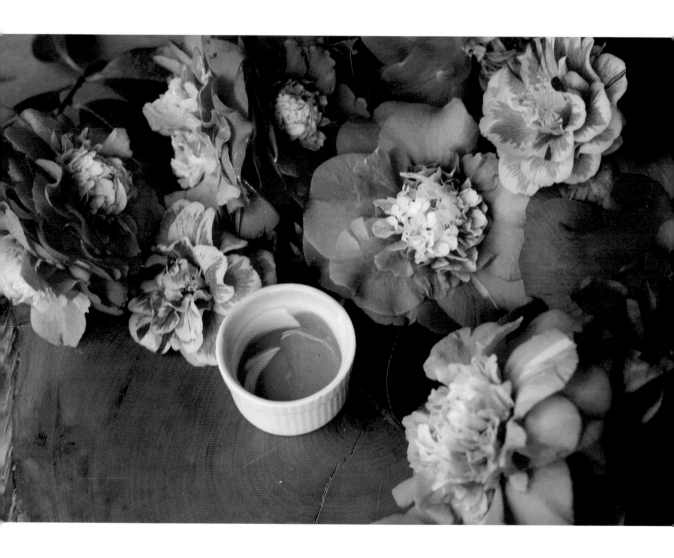

Green Goddess Facial Mask

One thing to remember for all your formulas using matcha: The higher quality the matcha, the better for your skin (and the better to drink!). The flowers and leaves surrounding this facial mask in the photo to the left are a variety of camellias.

2 ounces kaolin clay
1 ounce green clay
½ teaspoon matcha
½ teaspoon ground nettle leaf
½ teaspoon spirulina powder

Makes 4 ounces.

Mix all ingredients together, bottle, cap, and label. This recipe is a hefty dose of serious greens for your skin!

To use, blend a little of the mask with water in a separate mixing bowl, massage into face, let dry, and wash off. Follow with moisturizer.

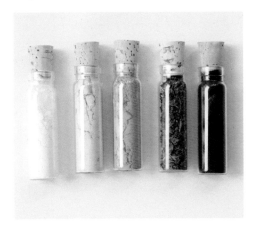

kaolin clay, bentonite clay, matcha, nettle leaf, spirulina powder

Matcha comes from the camellia plant; rather, camellia leaves are tea leaves. Green tea is steamed and dried leaves, oolong tea is mildly fermented, and black tea is fully fermented camellia leaves. Matcha, however, goes through a completely different process where, nearing harvest time, the leaves are covered so they get less and less sunlight. The finest matcha will have the brightest color. The amino acids in matcha create the savory (umami) flavor.

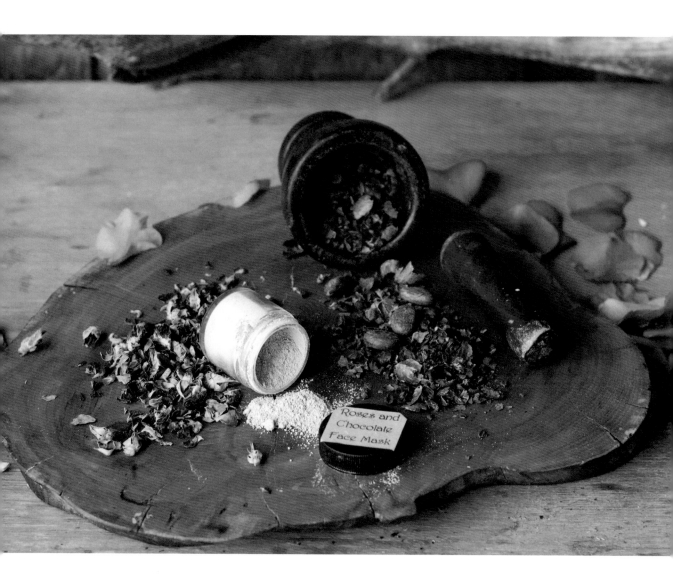

Roses and Chocolate Facial Mask

Irritation-reducing roses and antioxidant-packed chocolate make this facial mask a great blend for all skin types.

2 ounces kaolin clay
½ ounce bentonite
1 teaspoon cocoa powder
1 teaspoon rose powder

Makes 2¾ ounces.

Mix all ingredients together, bottle, cap, and label.

To use, blend a little of the mask with water in a separate mixing bowl, massage into face, let dry, and wash off. Follow with moisturizer.

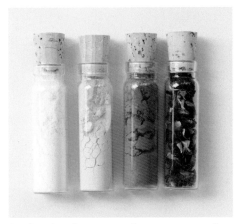

kaolin clay, bentonite clay, cocoa powder, rose petals

I think roses and chocolate are one of my favorite things to eat, drink, and rub all over my body, as well as share with my loved ones, so I couldn't help but add a mask with my favorite ingredients!

Illuminate Facial Mask

This facial mask is ideal for mature and dry skin types, helping to increase skin resiliency to external stressors such as sun, wind, oxygen, and gravity. With moisturizing marshmallow, nourishing chaga, circulation stimulating turmeric, fine line–reducing sandalwood, and healing vanilla, this is a precious blend of skin care ingredients.

½ cup garbanzo flour

½ cup kaolin clay

¼ cup bentonite clay

1 teaspoon sandalwood powder (spicatum)

¼ teaspoon turmeric

1 pinch powdered vanilla bean

¼ teaspoon ground chaga

1 teaspoon marshmallow root

Makes 1¼ cups.

Mix all ingredients together, bottle, and label.

To use, blend a little of the mask with water in a separate mixing bowl, massage into face, let dry, wash off, and follow with moisturizer.

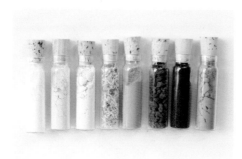

kaolin clay, bentonite clay, garbanzo flour, marshmallow root, sandalwood powder, chaga, vanilla bean powder, ground turmeric

This is very gentle and nourishing. Excellent for all skin types including mature, sensitive, and dry.

Toner/Hydrating Mists

Basic Toner

To tone and tame, to calm redness, irritations, puffy skin, or just because you like rose.

8 ounces rose hydrosol

Pour directly into a bottle with a spritzer attachment.

Use after washing face and before moisturizing, when you need a calm breath, when you're hot and bothered. . . . Seriously, I carry a bottle of this around with me during the summer to use all day long.

TONER PROMPT

As you will see, creating toners can be as easy or as complex as you choose to make them.

Try making rainbow toners, or mixing different tincture blends to get different colors and actions.

You can also add essential oils for skin type.

Queen of Hungary's Water I

Another type of toner—and possibly the first toner ever written about—is the cologne archetype Queen of Hungary's Water, which likely started with rosemary and other plants were added later. It was basically the elixir of longevity; it cured illness, kept skin youthful, and worked all sorts of magic.

8 ounces witch hazel
1 drop vetiver essential oil
2 drops sandalwood essential oil
½ drop patchouli essential oil
2 drops rose essential oil
1 drop orange blossom essential oil
2 drops lemon essential oil
2 drops lime essential oil
2 drops orange essential oil
3 drops lavender essential oil
3 drops rosemary essential oil

Makes about 8 ounces.

Blend all ingredients in a mason jar, cap, and shake. Pour into bottles with spritzer attachments.

To use, shake and then spray onto face, keeping out of eyes. Follow with moisturizer.

Queen of Hungary's Water II

This is my rendition of Queen of Hungary water, soaked in organic grape alcohol. The finished product smells so incredible that I use the straight stuff as perfume.

8 ounces organic grape alcohol*
1 teaspoon sandalwood powder
¼ teaspoon patchouli leaf
2 teaspoon rose buds
1 teaspoon orange blossoms
1 teaspoon dried lemon peel
1 teaspoon dried lime peel
1 teaspoon dried orange peel
1 teaspoon lavender
1 teaspoon rosemary

*I use a 190-proof variety from the Organic Alcohol Company.

Makes 8 ounces.

Put all ingredients in a jar with lid, shake 2 times daily for 2 weeks, strain through a coffee filter, and compost plant ingredients. Pour strained liquid into a bottle with spray attachment.

To use, add 1 ounce of tincture to 8 ounces of witch hazel.

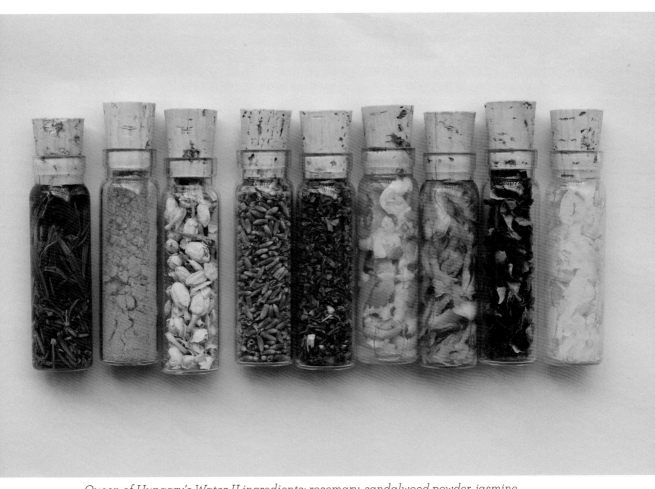

Queen of Hungary's Water II ingredients: rosemary, sandalwood powder, jasmine flowers, lavender, patchouli leaf, orange peel, lime peel, rose petals, lemon peel

Egyptian Eau de Toilette

This blend uses a variety of ingredients found in ancient Egypt. I like to think that the reason Egyptians were so good at embalming bodies to last forever was due to the ingredients they had on hand. It makes sense that it would help living skin keep its youth forever, as well.

8 ounces witch hazel

3 drops frankincense essential oil

1 drop jatamansi essential oil

2 drops benzoin essential oil

3 drops myrrh essential oil

1 drop galbanum essential oil

2 drops lotus essential oil

3 drops rose essential oil

1 drop cardamom essential oil

Makes 8 ounces.

Mix all ingredients together, shake well, and pour into bottles with spritzer attachments. Label.

To use, after washing face, spritz on toner, and follow with moisturizer.

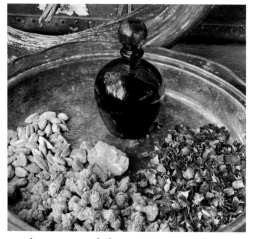

cardamom, myrrh, benzoin, rose petals

NOTES

Aqua Celestis

I created this recipe after I was inspired by a dream. This blend is used in many of the things I make. Although here we will use it as a toner, it works wonders for burns, cuts, abrasions, acne, scar reduction, wrinkle reduction— you name it. This is the water of miracles, but we will simply refer to it as the water of the heavens.

8 ounces witch hazel
1 ounce powdered myrrh
1 ounce powdered frankincense

Makes 8 ounces.

Blend all ingredients together in a jar with a sealed lid. Shake 2 times a day for 2 weeks. After this time, pour through a coffee filter into bottles with spritzer attachments. Label and enjoy.

To use, spritz onto clean face and follow with moisturizer, if you'd like. This stuff is so good for the skin that often I will not use a moisturizer with it.

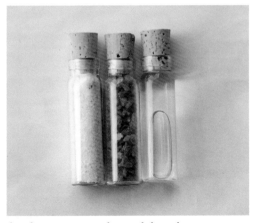

frankincense, myrrh, witch hazel

NOTES

Aqua Mellis

Honey has been used throughout history in many beauty formulations, and for good reason—it has many youth- and beauty-retaining qualities. In nature, honey never goes rancid, as it contains a host of antimicrobials and antifungals, not to mention it is antibacterial, antiseptic, and anti-inflammatory. It also contains probiotics. Imagine the potential this has for your skin! Perfection! Honey is moisturizing and softens the skin, reducing dryness and increasing plumpness. It has a plethora of wonderful enzymes that balance your complexion, too.

8 ounces water
½ teaspoon honey

Makes 8 ounces.

In a bowl, mix the ingredients together until honey is dissolved. Pour into bottles with spritzer attachment, label, and enjoy.

To use, wash and spray directly onto face. I like to spritz this on my face multiple times a day.

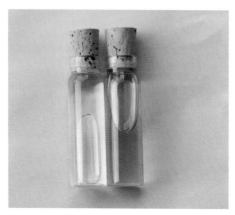

water, honey

Keep in mind this mist will go rancid now that you've added water to the honey. So keep this mix in the refrigerator and use within a month.

Siren's Blend Toner

This recipe smells so divine it may as well be the aroma of the siren's song, so intoxicating it has created many, many addicted users, transporting the wearer to a magical ocean retreat, while being incredibly soothing for the skin.

4 ounces rose hydrosol

4 ounces orange blossom hydrosol

3 drops seaweed tincture

$1/8$ teaspoon sea salt

Makes 8 ounces.

Place all ingredients in a bottle with a lid. Shake until well incorporated. Pour into a bottle with a sprizter attachment and label.

To use, wash face and spritz on toner, being careful of the eyes. Follow with moisturizer.

NOTES

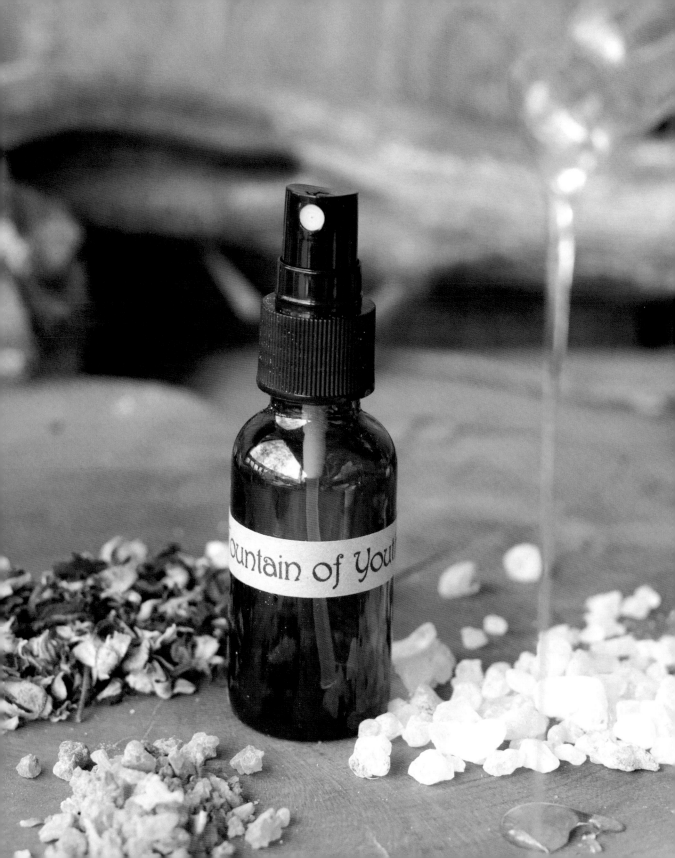

Fountain of Youth

This is a blend of all the wonderful above ingredients, but the coolest thing about this blend is it's truly for your whole body (on the outside anyway). This formula is as incredible for the hair as it is for the sensitive facial skin, but don't stop there—apply it to your whole body! I'm not kidding, I like to generously spray this all over myself after a shower, then follow with moisturizer.

4 ounces Aqua Celestis, filtered (page 73)
4 ounces rose hydrosol
½ teaspoon honey

Makes 8 ounces.

Place all ingredients in a container with a lid, shake well, and pour into bottles with spritzer attachments. Label and then store in the refrigerator.

Due to the honey mixed with liquid in this blend, it has the potential to turn rancid, so add a preservative, like a tiny 3-milliliter shot of alcohol, or keep in the fridge.

NOTES

....
....
....
....
....
....
....
....
....

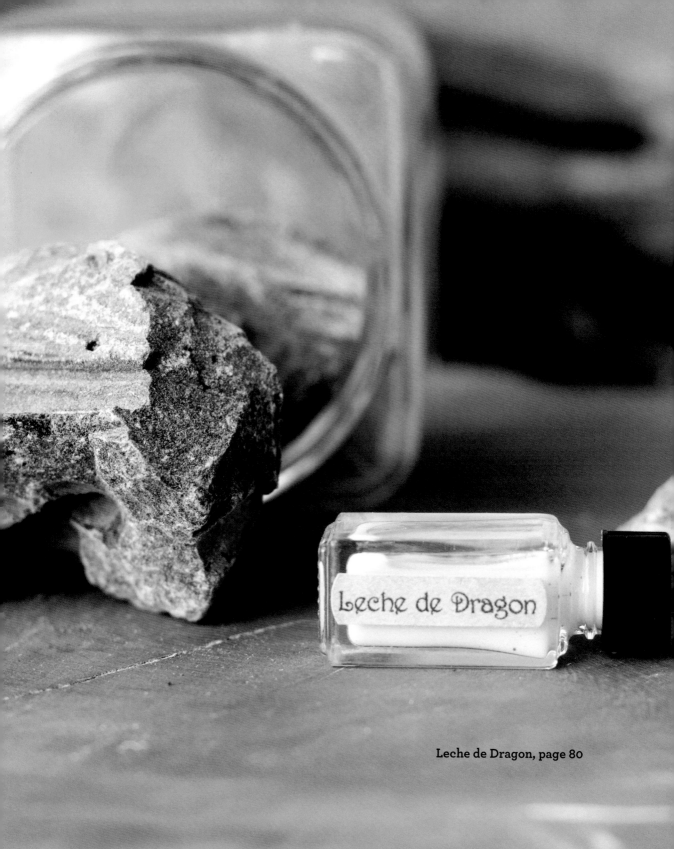

Leche de Dragon, page 80

Blemish Reducers

A NOTE ABOUT BLEMISH REDUCERS

Blemish reducers are generally used after a good face washing but can really be applied any time you feel the need for a quick spot reduction.

These work on acne, black heads, white heads, and inflammations. They are comprised of strong astringents and bacteria slayers, are antifungal, and they increase healing while creating a pH balance uninhabitable by irritating microbes.

While toners work to all over balance and tone, they are not as strong of an astringent or drying agent as a blemish reducer, so while these are definitely not something you would want all over your face on healthy skin, they are highly effective for spot reduction and maintaining skin mantle harmony.

A note on alcohol in skin care (as blemish reducers generally contain a high percent): alcohol may be not so good for the skin because it's stressful, but it helps aid in rapid absorption of nutrients, tightening skin, cleaning skin, destroying bad bacteria, and it can work as a preservative. So use it sparingly, but don't be afraid to use it if the benefits outweigh the detriment. With natural skin care, you're automatically doing more good than bad with well-formulated recipes.

Leche de Dragon

A powerful blemish-reducing recipe that uses the superb healing and blood-cleansing attributes of dragon's blood resin and a gentle drop of humectant agave. I created this recipe for my two teenage children who recently started breaking out here and there; they were begging for something to cure their blemishes overnight. This liquid turns from blood red to a milky red when finished; it's really fun to make!

½ ounce dragon's blood tincture
¼ cup witch hazel
1 teaspoon agave
3 drops tea tree oil
3 drops rosewood leaf oil

Makes about ¼ cup.

Strain dragon's blood tincture following instructions on page 21.

Blend all ingredients together, shake well, bottle, and label. Blemish reducers can be stored in air-tight jars like mason jars or in easy-to-use smaller bottles with spritzer tops.

Apply to blemishes as needed.

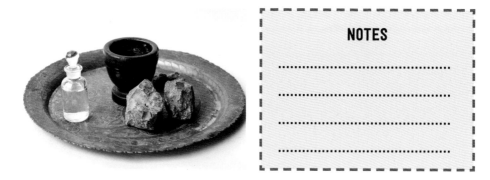

NOTES

....

....

....

....

Queen of Hungary's Blemish Reducer

¼ cup witch hazel
½ ounces Queen of Hungary's Water II (page 70)

Makes ¼ cup.

Mix ingredients together well, bottle, and label. Blemish reducers can be stored in airtight jars like mason jars or in easy-to-use smaller bottles with spritzer tops.

Apply to blemishes as needed.

· ·

Quick Blemish Reducer

Frankincense and myrrh, being the sap or blood of the tree, act to purify and heal our blood by fighting off bacteria and increasing cellular turnover.

¼ cup alcohol
5 drops myrrh essential oil
5 drops frankincense essential oil

Makes ¼ cup.

Mix all ingredients together and shake well. Blemish reducers can be stored in air-tight jars like mason jars or in easy-to-use smaller bottles with spritzer tops.

Use on blemishes as needed.

BLEMISH REDUCER PROMPT

Substitute an alternative herbal tincture, or try adding a few essential oils. Switch it up; there are many wonderful astringent herbs and essential oils.

NOTES

· ·

· ·

· ·

· ·

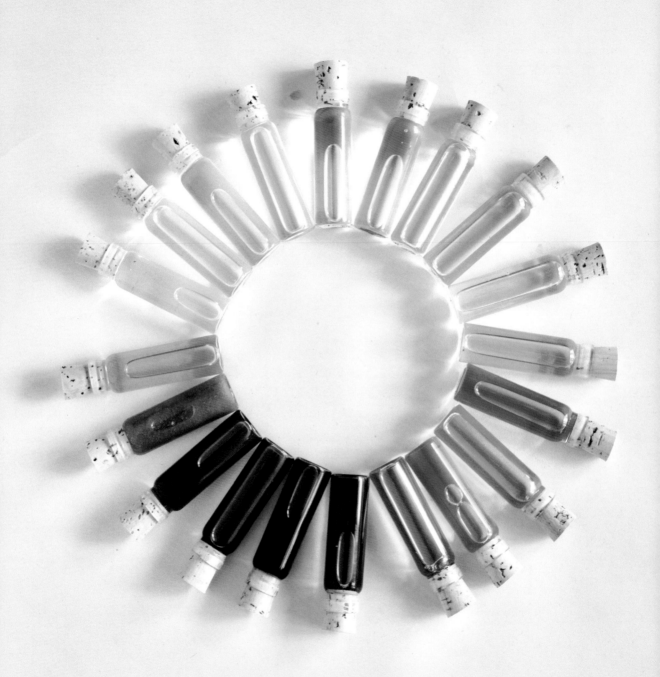

Facial Moisturizers

Basic Face Moisturizer

This moisturizer is not too heavy, is healing and nourishing, yet incredibly simple and can be easily varied with additions of essential oils or herbal oil extracts (see page 22).

1 ounce squalene

1 ounce apricot kernel oil

1 ounce jojoba oil

2 drops jasmine sambac

Makes about 3 ounces.

Blend all ingredients together, mixing thoroughly. Bottle in a container with a dropper top.

To use, take drop 3 to 8 drops in palms of hands and rub into face in outward circular motions.

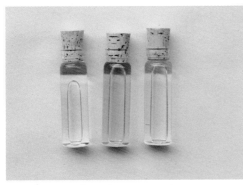

Squalene, jojoba oil, apricot oil

NOTES

....

....

....

....

....

Acne and Oily–Prone Skin Moisturizer

The beauty of this moisturizer is that it is low on the comedogenic scale, astringent, and moisturizing without being greasy. It tightens pores and cleanses the face with a bacteria-slaying blend of essential oils.

2 ounces hazelnut oil

3 drops black cumin oil

1 gram carrot seed oil

2 grams rosehip seed oil

2 grams black raspberry seed oil

1 gram castor oil

4 drops cypress essential oil

6 drops myrrh essential oil

1 drop frankincense essential oil

8 drops lavender essential oil

1 drop chamomile essential oil

5 drops bergapten-free bergamot essential oil

Makes 2¼ ounces.

Blend all ingredients together. I like to shake them in a jar for extra mixing.

Pour into applicator jar with pump and label.

To use, after spritzing toner on face, rub about three drops of oil between palms, and work into facial skin. Enjoy your magical skin!

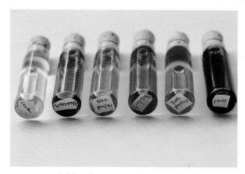

castor oil, black cumin, black raspberry, hazelnut, rosehip seed, carrot

NOTES

Sensitive Mature Dry Skin Moisturizer

This blend contains the beautiful camellia plant oil. It's actually the plant that the tea comes from. Camellia is phenomenal for the skin, highly nourishing, reduces fine lines and wrinkles, and is non-greasy. This magical blend is made with a number of other supportive oils and the outcome is simply divine!

3 ounces camellia oil

1 gram pomegranate oil

1 gram borage oil

1 gram meadowfoam oil

1 gram indigo naturalis oil extraction (see page 22)

2 ounces apricot oil

1 ounce squalene

8 drops sandalwood essential oil

Makes 6¼ ounces.

Blend all ingredients together. I like to shake them in a jar for extra mixing.

Pour into applicator jar with pump and label.

To use, after spritzing toner on face, rub about three drops of oil between palms, and work into facial skin. Enjoy your magical skin!

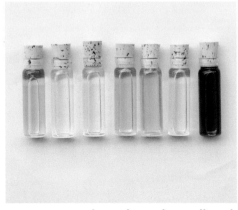

pomegranate oil, squalene oil, camellia oil, meadow foam oil, apricot oil, borage oil, indigo oil

NOTES

....

....

....

....

....

....

....

Solid Facial Moisturizer

This is a basic moisturizing recipe taking the idea of liquid oils and making a rich, solid stick that is easy to apply. This is a good recipe to play around with by substituting varying oils and butters to get a moisturizer that works perfectly for you.

10 grams sal butter

10 grams cocoa butter

5 grams beeswax

¼ gram argan oil

¼ gram jojoba oil

¼ gram rose hip seed oil

¾ gram evening primrose oil

½ gram apricot kernel oil

1 drop jasmine sambac

This recipe makes enough to fill 5 to 6 lip balm tubes.

Melt butters and wax together over double boiler and then remove from heat. Add oils, including essential oil, and mix well. Pour carefully into lip balm tubes.

Let cool to room temp, cap, label, and use often!

To use, apply just a touch of moisturizer to face as needed and rub in.

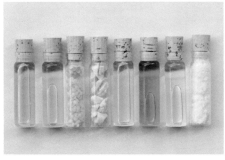

jojoba oil, argan oil, beeswax pastilles, cocoa butter, apricot oil, rosehip oil, evening primrose oil, sal butter

FACIAL MOISTURIZER PROMPT
Try mixing your own facial stick just for your skin with different oils and butters—just make sure the amount of oils equals 2.25 grams and the butters equal 20 grams. Try using a different essential oil, just for you.

EYES & EARS

The skin around the eyes is some of the most sensitive and thinnest skin on our bodies. The eyes can get easily irritated and are greatly affected by heat, so it's super important that *you* stay hydrated so *they* stay hydrated.

I like to keep a spritzer of rose hydrosol next to my computer to spritz my eyes whenever I start feeling fatigue creep up, if I start getting blinky because they are dry, tired, etc. Cucumber slices over eyes are always wonderful, too—they are moisturizing, cooling, regenerative to the skin and also help reduce bags and minimize wrinkles.

For many of us, sometimes bags or dark circles around eyes may be an issue. To reduce this, it's good to introduce circulation-enhancing ingredients as well as tightening and toning astringents.

Witch hazel is great for this, but keep it out of the eyes. Castor oil and hazelnut oil are astringent oils while apricot kernel oil is extremely gentle and works wonders to reduce wrinkles.

In the morning, I like to spritz my eyes with rose hydrosol, do some eye exercises, such as looking all the way to each side, gently at first and then as far as I can next, followed by looking up and looking down, then some eye circles. All very gently.

I also like to eat fruits and veggies to nourish my eyes from the inside. I am careful about what I let in, and I abstain from television and brutality, avoid the news, and spend a lot of time in nature, creating art and being with beautiful humans. Always be mindful of what you let into your sight, for you digest what you see as well as what you eat. Remember the saying *you are what you eat*? Well, *you are what you see* can apply here, too. What are you letting into your vision?

Simple Eye Moisturizer | 90
Rejuvenative Daily Eye Serum | 91
Evening Eyes Serum | 92
Eyebrow Oil | 93
Eyebrow Balm | 94
Ear Anointing Oil | 95

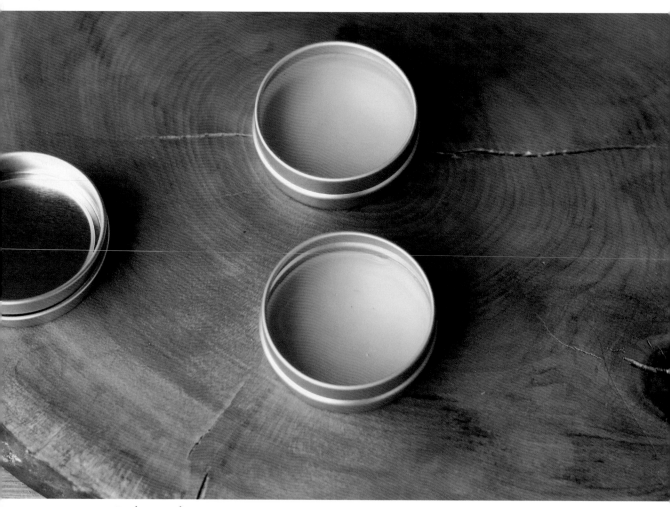

Eyebrow Balm, page 94

Applying Products

To get the most out of applying hydration around the eye area, massage products around eyes, with little circles moving from near the eye out, always pulling in the direction of the ear. Finish with massaging from the inside next to the nose to the outside of eye area across the cheek bone and down to the neck by the lymph nodes. This will aid the skin's removal of excess toxins and fluids around the eye area and into the lymphatic system. This will reduce bags, dark circles, and general puffiness.

Serums versus Moisturizers

Moisturizers do just that: moisturize. While they can also have excess nutrients, their prime purpose is to moisturize. Serums, on the other hand, are a potent blend of powerful and often highly concentrated ingredients, kind of like a supplement for the skin. Serums can be layered with moisturizers or used alone.

Simple Eye Moisturizer

This is the ideal blend if you want to keep eye moisturizing simple yet effective.

8 grams apricot kernal oil
8 grams squalene
1 drop jasmine sambac (optional)

Makes 16 grams.

Mix all ingredients in a little half-ounce jar with dropper, shake, and label.

To use, massage 2 to 3 drops around eyes. Finish with massaging from the inside next to nose to the outside of eye area, across the cheek bone, and down to the neck by the lymph nodes.

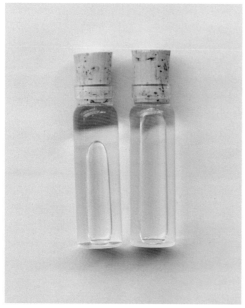

squalene oil, apricot kernel oil

NOTES

....

....

....

....

....

....

....

....

....

Rejuvenate Daily Eye Serum

This blend is a wonderful way to start the day around the sensitive eye area. It contains a potent package of fine line and wrinkle repelling, tightening, and soothing herbal oils and precious essential oils revered for their youth enhancing qualities.

6 grams jojoba oil

2 grams argan oil

2 grams camellia oil

1 gram pomegranate oil

1 gram rosehip seed oil

1 gram raspberry seed oil

10 drops carrot seed oil

2 drops sandalwood essential oil

1 drop myrrh essential oil

1 drop immortelle essential oil

Makes ½ ounce.

Mix all ingredients in a little jar with dropper, shake, and label.

To use, massage 2 to 3 drops around eyes. Finish by massaging from the inside next to nose to the outside of eye area, across the cheek bone, and down to the neck by the lymph nodes.

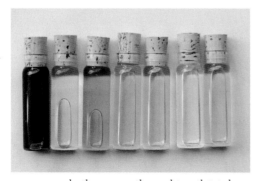

carrot seed oil, argan oil, rosehip oil, jojoba oil, pomegranate oil, camellia oil, raspberry oil

NOTES

....

....

....

....

....

Evening Eyes Serum

Wake up refreshed with healthy, lovely eyes! This serum has a bit heavier feel due to the castor oil and will sit on the skin longer than a day moisturizer. The blend is also astringent so it will moisturize and tighten and tone skin.

2 ounces castor oil

3 grams green tea (matcha) oil extract in grapeseed oil (see page 22)

3 grams oregon grape root oil extract in olive oil (see page 22)

2 drops blue yarrow essential oil

2 drops frankincense essential oil

2 drops cypress oil

Makes a little over 2 ounces.

Mix all ingredients in a little jar with dropper, shake, and label.

To use, massage 2 to 3 drops around eyes. Finish with massaging from the inside next to nose to the outside of eye area, across the cheek bone, and down to the neck by the lymph nodes.

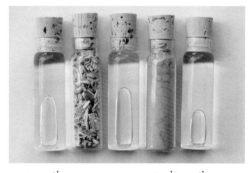

castor oil, oregon grape root, olive oil, matcha, grapeseed oil

NOTES

....

....

....

....

....

Eyebrow Oil

This oil helps add a bit of shine, nourishment, and can help increase thickness and overall brow health.

6 grams apricot oil
½ grams castor oil
½ grams bhringaraj oil extract in grapeseed oil (see page 22)
½ grams horsetail oil extract in olive oil (see page 22)
½ grams nettle oil extract in olive oil (see page 22)
½ gram raspberry oil
2 drops sandalwood essential oil

Makes 8.5 grams.

Mix all ingredients in a little jar with dropper, shake, and label.

To use, massage 1 to 3 drops per eyebrow, rubbing oil into brow and then smoothing it down and shaping it.

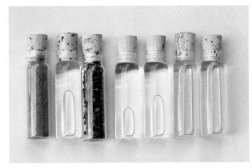

bhringaraj powder, horsetail oil, nettle leaf, grapeseed oil, castor oil, apricot kernel oil, raspberry seed oil, olive oil

NOTES

....

....

....

....

....

Eyebrow Balm

This conditioning blend works to hold brows in place without being greasy. Use eyebrow balm in the morning along with your regular skin care routine to keep the brows in place all day long.

10 grams coconut oil
10 grams jojoba oil
5 grams beeswax
1 drops myrrh essential oil
1 drop jasmine sambac
3 drops bergamot bergaptene-free essential oil

This recipe makes almost 1 ounce of eyebrow balm and is pictured on page 88.

Measure oils and beeswax into a heatproof container, set over double boiler on medium heat, and stir until melted. Remove from heat, add essential oils, mix well, pour into tins, cap when set, and label.

To use, rub a wee bit into finger and thumb and stroke into eyebrows in the direction of the hair. Work into eyebrows and shape them as desired.

NOTES

This conditioning blend works to hold brows in place without being greasy.

Ear Anointing Oil

Ears are an often forgotten area when it comes to skin care, but being that they are full of nerve endings, help us hear, and are an undeniably important part of our whole body system, they also need to be treated with care. Simply massaging the ears daily is important and can be linked to myriad healthy benefits. If you want to learn more about how beneficial it is to massage the ears, do a search on reflexology.

1 ounce jojoba oil
1 ounce sunflower oil
½ ounce borage oil
5 drops sea buckthorn berry oil
3 drops rosemary essential oil

Makes 2½ ounces.

Mix all ingredients together, bottle, and label.

To use, massage about 2 to 3 drops onto ears. Start with the top of the ear and massage down to the bottom, massage around the cartilage on the inside, and end lightly by pinching the ear from the top to the bottom and around the cartilage on the inside.

NOTES

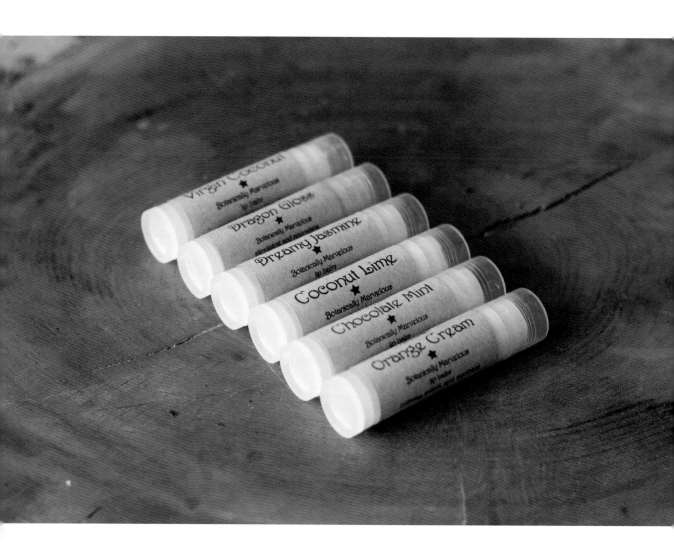

96

LIPS

In this short section, I've included a few recipes to get you started on lip basics with polishes or buffs to remove dead skin cells and moisturize the skin underneath, followed by a variety of wonderful lip balms.

The lip polishes and buffs are super simple, highly effective, and you can eat them. Really. Skin food. To use any lip polish, simply lick your lips and rub a bit of lip buff on them. Then rub lips together, lick sugar off, and follow with lip balm. The key to perfection with crafting these is to avoid using too much oil or they will separate, but if you have too little oil, the blend will be hard and not creamy. We're aiming for a perfect creamy and easily applicable blend for the buffs and polishes.

The lip balms are recipes for perfectly kissable lips! The Chocolate Mint Lip Balm on page 100 is a super simple lip balm recipe that uses just five ingredients. It's effective for soft, kissable lips and a wonderful daily protector from dry, chapped lips. Prompts for these recipes add a pretty little twist to the basic formula that you'll enjoy!

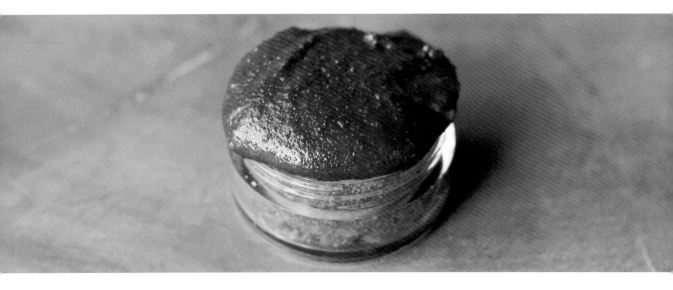

Chocolate Lip Buff

Chocolate is super nourishing for the skin and packed with antioxidants, which makes this lip buff a great addition to your lip care routine.

0.4 ounce cocoa butter
1¹/₅ ounces jojoba oil
4 grams castor sugar*
¹/₃ ounce cocoa powder (less or more depending upon how chocolatey you like it)

Makes 5½ ounces.

Weigh out cocoa butter and jojoba oil in heatproof container, and melt over double boiler. Remove from heat, add in powdered ingredients, and mix well. Pour into container, cap, and label.

To use, lick lips, rub in a bit of polish with your finger, rub your lips together, lick off, follow with lip balm.

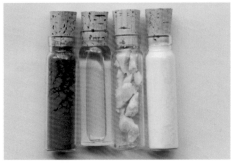

cocoa powder, jojoba oil, cocoa butter, castor sugar

To make your own castor sugar, take regular sugar and put in blender until super fine but not yet powdered sugar, or purchase castor sugar from the store.

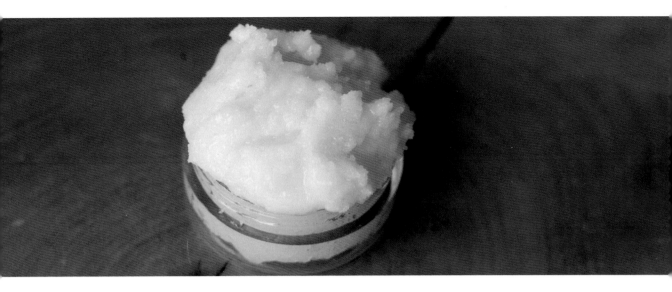

Vanilla Lip Buff

Simple, sweet, and effective, vanilla makes this recipe smell and taste like cake frosting.

1½ ounces jojoba oil
4 ounces castor sugar
1 pinch ground vanilla

Makes 5½ ounces.

Weigh out jojoba oil, add in powdered ingredients, and mix well. Pour into container, cap, and label.

To use, lick lips, rub in a bit of polish with your finger, rub your lips together, lick off, and follow with lip balm.

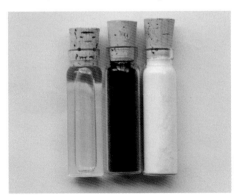

jojoba oil, vanilla bean powder, castor sugar

Learn how to make your own castor sugar at home on page 98. But feel free to use store-bought if you'd like.

Chocolate Mint Lip Balm

This is my personal favorite lip balm of all time. It also makes your lips smell very fresh!

7 grams beeswax
20 grams sunflower oil
12 grams cocoa butter
1 tiny pinch organic stevia, if you want a touch of sweet
7 drops peppermint essential oil

This recipe creates enough to fill 7 lip balm tubes.

Weigh all ingredients, except peppermint, in a heatproof glass measuring cup.

Place your cooking pan on the burner and fill with enough water to be equal with the materials in your glass heatproof cup.

Turn burner to medium heat, place heatproof cup into water bath, stir ingredients until melted, then remove from heat and wipe water off bottom of glass cup. Add peppermint if desired, and mix.

Pour into lip balm tubes. The stevia will have settled in the bottom of your heatproof cup, so simply stop pouring into lip balm tubes once you notice the liquid gets grainy and toss what's left. Your lip balm will still be sweet, don't worry!

Let cool until solidified. Cap the tubes and label your balm. Use for yourself or make gifts!

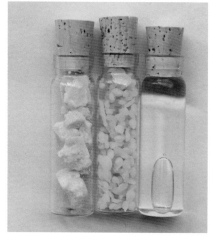

cocoa butter, beeswax pastilles, sunflower oil

LIP BALM PROMPTS

Check out these substitutions!

Jasmine Twist
Substitute the peppermint for 3 drops jasmine.

Orange Cream
Substitute the peppermint essential oil for orange essential oil.

Now prompt yourself to come up with something that goes well with vanilla or cocoa for a delightful lip balm recipe all your own!

Virgin Coconut Lip Balm

This sweet and basic coconut lip balm is an easy recipe to add different essential oils to create a wide variety of flavored lip balms.

12 grams beeswax
12 grams organic shea butter
25 grams coconut oil
1 pinch stevia, if you want it sweet

This recipe will fill about 12 lip balm tubes.

Weigh all ingredients in a heatproof glass measuring cup.

Place your cooking pan on the burner and fill with enough water to be equal with the materials in your glass heatproof cup.

Turn burner to medium heat, place heatproof cup into water bath, and stir ingredients until melted. Remove from heat, wipe water off bottom of glass cup, and mix.

Pour into lip balm tubes. The stevia will have settled in the bottom of your heatproof cup, so simply stop pouring into lip balm tubes once you see that it is grainy and toss the rest. Your lip balm will still be sweet, don't worry!

Let cool until solidified. Cap the tubes and label your balm. Use for yourself or give as gifts!

NOTES

....

....

....

....

....

LIP BALM PROMPT

Try this tropical twist!

Virgin Coconut and Lime
Simply add about 6 drops of lime essential oil for a tropical twist.

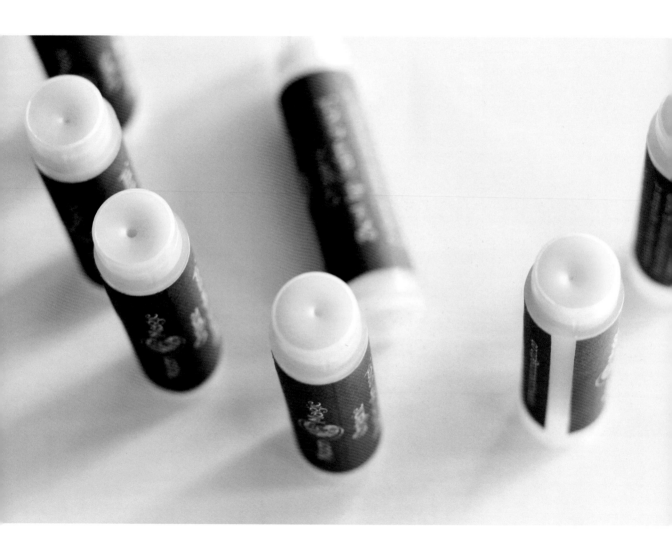

Best Lip Balm Ever

This special recipe is really packed with lip nourishing oils, it is very soothing and healing.

5 grams coconut oil

12 grams mango butter

5 grams almond oil

14 grams jojoba oil

$\frac{1}{8}$ teaspoon sea buckthorn berry oil (too much will dye your skin)

12 grams beeswax

3 drops lavender essential oil

3 drops sandalwood essential oil

This recipe will fill about 12 lip balm tubes.

Weigh all ingredients in a heatproof glass measuring cup.

Place your cooking pan on the burner and fill with enough water to be equal with the materials in your glass heatproof cup.

Turn burner to medium heat, place heatproof cup into water bath, and stir ingredients until melted. Remove from heat, wipe water off bottom of glass cup, and mix.

Pour into lip balm tubes.

Let cool until solidified. Cap the tubes and label your balm. Use for yourself or give as gifts!

NOTES

....

....

....

....

....

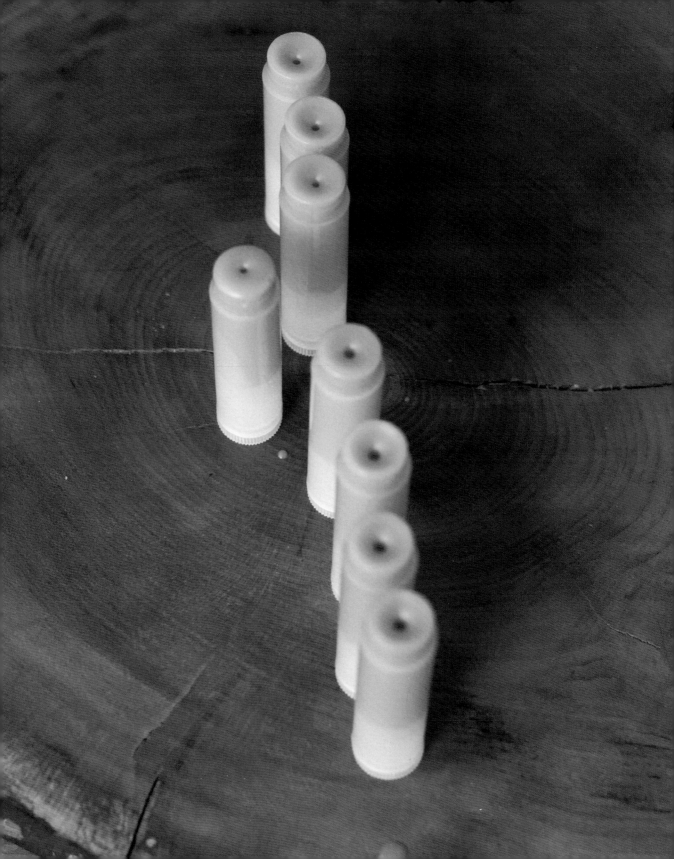

Lip Plumping Solid Gloss

Castor oil creates a glossy look on lips, while the cinnamon draws and stimulates the blood flow, enhancing soft, warm, plump, beautiful lips.

18 grams castor oil
12 grams mango butter
12 grams beeswax
1 pinch super finely powdered dragon's blood resin, if desired
1 tiny pinch stevia, if you want it sweet
6 drops cinnamon bark essential oil

This recipe will fill about 12 lip balm tubes.

Weigh all ingredients, except cinnamon, in a heatproof glass measuring cup.

Place your cooking pan on the burner and fill with enough water to be equal with the materials in your glass heatproof cup.

Turn burner to medium heat, place heatproof cup into water bath, and stir ingredients until melted. Remove from heat, wipe water off bottom of glass cup, add cinnamon, and mix.

Pour into lip balm tubes. The stevia will have settled in the bottom of your heatproof cup, so simply stop pouring into lip balm tubes once the liquid gets grainy and toss what remains. Your lip balm will still be sweet, don't worry!

Let cool until solidified. Cap the tubes and label your balm. Use for yourself or gift to someone you love!

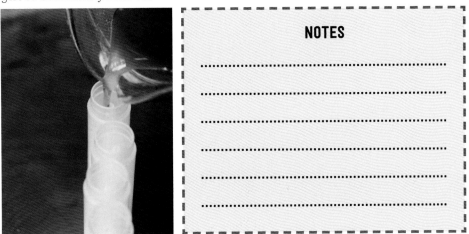

NOTES

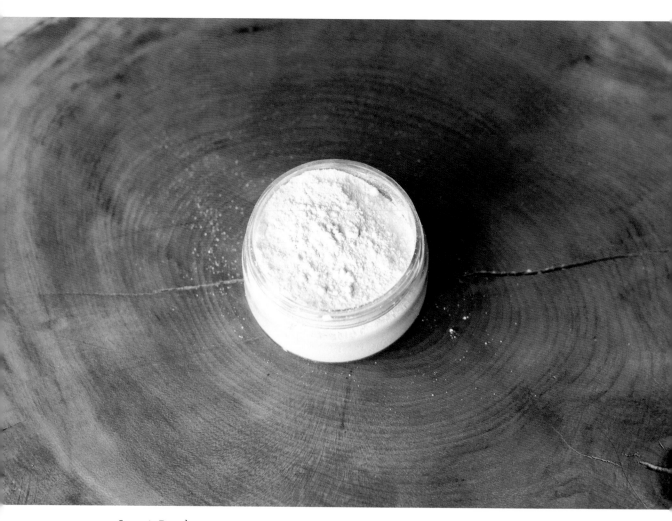

Armpit Powder, page 108

ARMPITS

Armpits are a wonderful thing to care for—smelling great around other people is a good idea to maintain friendships and healthy work environments. The following recipes are wonderful natural blends that keep bacteria at a minimum and absorb sweat. However, they are not antiperspirant recipes; sweating is a really important thing to allow your body to do and antiperspirants are, in my opinion and many others', just chemical cakes.

Armpit Powder

(Deodorant Powder Base)

If you like a gentle dusting of the armpits rather than rubbing in a solid, this is for you. This powder is also the base for the rest of the solid deodorant recipes. If you are sensitive to baking soda, simply omit it.

1 tablespoon baking soda
1 tablespoon arrowroot powder
1 tablespoon kaolin clay

Makes ¼ cup.

Mix all ingredients together well. Pour into your container of choice.

To use, pat a little powder onto armpits as needed. Rub in until fully incorporated with skin to avoid white spots on clothes.

NOTES

....

....

....

ARMPIT PROMPT
Try adding a few essential oils or powdered frankincense and myrrh into your mix for aromatic enhancement and bacteria-slaying potential.

Armpit Spritz

If you like spray-on deodorant, this blend does the trick.

3 ounces aqua celestis (page 73)
4 drops lemongrass oil

Makes 3 ounces.

Pour all into bottle with a spritzer top and label.

To use, shake spritz and then spray onto armpits as needed.

Deodorant Cream

Using the base mix in the previous recipe, this recipe incorporates plant butters and oils for a smooth, creamy deodorant application that goes on comfortably and can last all day.

½ ounce shea butter
½ ounce sal butter
½ ounce grapeseed oil
10 drops essential oil of choice
1 ounce deodorant base powder (see page 108)

Makes 2½ ounces.

Weigh out butters and grapeseed oil into heatproof mixing bowl, set over double boiler until melted, and remove from heat. Add essential oils to your melted mixture and blend.

Next, add your deodorant base powder and whisk in until no clumps remain. Scoop into jars, cap, and label.

To use, take a pea-sized amount of deodorant cream onto your finger tips and rub into each armpit until you can no longer see it.

NOTES

DEODORANT FORMULATING PROMPT
Using the basic deodorant cream recipe, substitute an oil blend of your own, weighing a total of ½ ounce. Use different butters if you choose, as long as it equals 1 ounce total weight. Create an essential oil blend that not only smells good but slays bacteria.

Teenage Armpit Angst

This recipe is a spin-off of the Deodorant Cream recipe (page 109), but uses a variety of oils known for their bacteria-slaying benefits as well as a specifically formulated aromatic blend.

½ gram cranberry seed oil
½ gram meadowfoam seed oil
½ gram black currant oil
⅔ gram rosehip seed oil
1 gram jojoba oil
2 grams dragon's blood oil extraction (see page 22)
10 grams grapeseed oil
25 grams shea butter
5 drops scent blend
5–10 drops essential oils of choice
1 ounce Armpit Powder (page 108)

Makes 1½ ounces.

Weigh out oil and butter into heatproof mixing bowl, set over double boiler until melted, and remove from heat. Add essential oils to your melted mixture and blend. Next, add your armpit powder and whisk in until no clumps remain. Scoop into jars, cap, and label.

To use, take a pea-sized amount of deodorant cream onto your fingertips and rub into each armpit until you can no longer see it.

NOTES

My friend's teenage daughter found herself needing to apply deodorant multiple times a day and was simply embarrassed. She wanted a deodorant that would work all day with one application.

I formulated this recipe and my friend's daughter tested it; it worked all day long, including all throughout volleyball practice. One application in the morning was all she needed.

HANDS

We use our hands all day long for everything. Caring for these wonderful parts of our being is so important. This section includes recipes to help maintain and repair happy healthy hands. These recipes can be used by themselves but also make for a very nice hand massage session. Start with the Coffee Sugar Scrub (on page 133) to exfoliate dry skin and follow with the Cuticle Cream on page 112. Then you could fill in exceptionally dry rough spots with the Cracks and Chaps Balm (page 116) and finish by massaging in Hand Butter (page 115).

Cuticle Cream

The featured cuticle cream is a sweet, easy, and incredibly helpful thing, excellent for hangnails and cuticles.

15 grams shea butter

5 grams beeswax

5 grams cocoa butter

7 grams mango butter

10 grams nettle herbal oil (see page 22)

3 drops lemon essential oil

3 drops myrrh essential oil

10 grams arrowroot powder

This recipe will fill 3 to 4 half-ounce tins.

Weigh out shea, beeswax, cocoa, mango, and nettle oil in a heatproof container. Set over double boiler until melted. Remove from heat, add essential oils and arrowroot, and mix until fully incorporated. Pour into half-ounce tins, let set, cap, and label.

To use, take a small amount of cuticle cream and work into cuticles and over nail and around fingertip area, softening the area. Re-apply as often as desired.

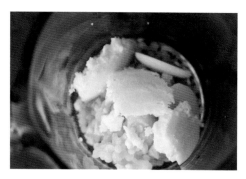

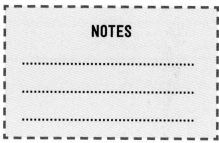

NOTES

....

....

....

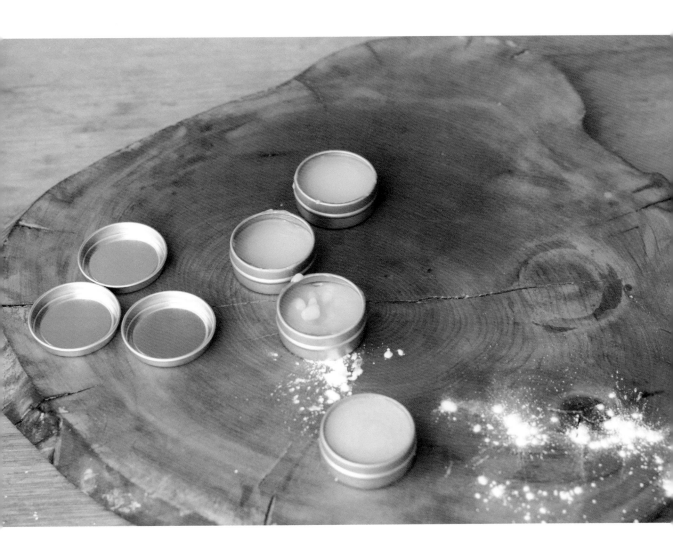

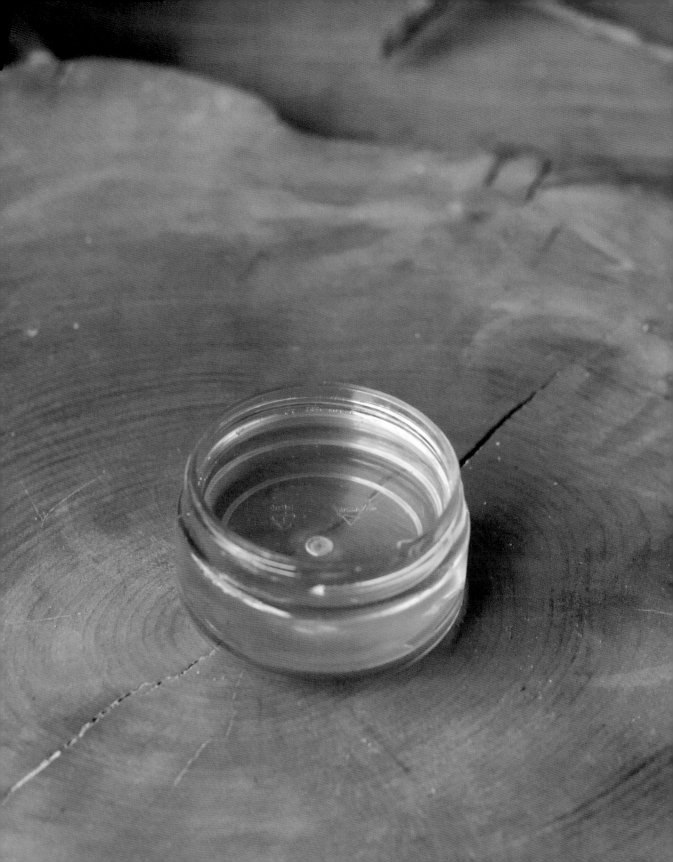

Hand Butter

This recipe is perfect for softening the hands and works really well for extremely dry skin, cracks, and rough spots.

1 ounce shea butter
1 ounce cocoa butter
1 ounce mango butter
$^1/_5$ ounces jojoba oil
5–10 drops lavender essential oil

Makes about 3 ounces.

Weigh out shea, cocoa, mango, and jojoba oil in a heatproof container. Set over double boiler until melted. Remove from heat, add essential oil, and mix until fully incorporated. Pour into 1-ounce tins or pans, let set, cap, and label.

To use, take a small amount of hand butter and work into hands, and re-apply as often desired.

NOTES

....
....
....
....
....
....

HAND BUTTER PROMPT

What other oils, essential oils, or herbal oils could you substitute in this recipe for specific hand needs?

Cracks and Chaps Balm

This recipe utilizes the powers of a particularly potent tri-force of skin-knitting herbs: comfrey, yarrow, and dragon's blood resin.

12 grams shea butter

5 grams olive oil

12 grams beeswax

1 pinch dragon's blood resin, ultra-fine powdered

10 grams comfrey herbal oil (see page 22)

10 grams yarrow herbal oil (see page 22)

3 drops cypress essential oil

3 drops eucalyptus essential oil

3 drops rosemary essential oil

This recipe makes enough balm to fill 3 to 4 half-ounce tins.

Place shea butter, olive oil, beeswax, and dragon's blood resin into heatproof container and set over double boiler until melted and dragon's blood resin is well incorporated. Remove from heat, add comfrey and yarrow—reheat if it starts to set up too quickly. Add essential oils. Pour into tins, allow to set, cap, and label.

To use, apply generously as needed to any area with particularly dry skin, cracks, or chaps, but keep out of open wounds.

NOTES

....

....

....

....

....

....

Comfrey is an herb that works to knit skin back together; it works really, really well, so be certain your hands are clean before you use it. Yarrow enhances the circulatory powers of comfrey, and dragon's blood resin moves the blood and cleanses it, and keeps out bacteria as well.

BODY

This section offers a variety of recipes to heal and nourish your entire body.

We start with dusting powders, for those of us who aren't into oil-based moisturizers. These will include arrowroot powder. Arrowroot is skin softening and was used historically to pull toxins out of arrow wounds and heal skin. It absorbs excess oil and draws moisture onto the skin.

The mists in this section are pleasantly hydrating blends to be spritzed on the skin whenever needed, just like the facial mists/toners we made earlier.

Finally, we wrap up with body oils. Im a big fan of using body oil over lotions for moisturizing; oils penetrate skin quicker than lotions. While you can use most oils to moisturize the skin, some are definitely better than others. Depending on what season it is, you may wish to vary what you use on your skin, such as heavier oils for dry winter skin and lighter oils for warm (prone to sweating) summer skin.

Dusting Powders

For soft skin, these are perfect for those who don't like moisturizers such as lotions. Dusting powders help keep skin silky smooth.

Basic Dusting Powder

Arrowroot powder (desired amount)

Simply sprinkle arrowroot onto skin, and rub all over. That's it! (You can put it in a cute bottle if you want to for daily use.)

. . . .

Herbal Dusting Powder

1 cup arrowroot powder
3 tablespoons dried lavender flowers
1 tablespoon dried chamomile flowers

Makes 1 cup.

Mix ingredients together, put in sealed jar, shake, and set aside for one week, shaking daily. You can choose to leave the flowers in or strain them out. If you're leaving the flowers in, place the powder in a jar with a shaker top to keep the flowers inside when you sprinkle the powder.

HERBAL DUSTING POWDER PROMPT
Create your own blend of dried herbs to use instead of lavender and chamomile to care for your skin specifically, or just to smell incredible.

To use, sprinkle powder all over the body and rub into your skin.

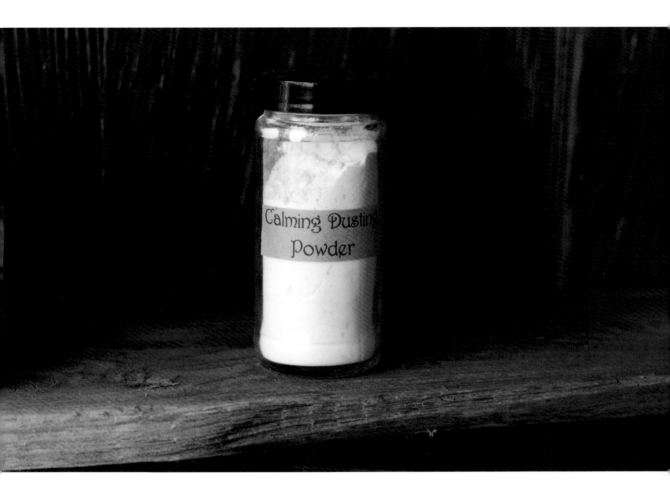

Calming Dusting Powder

6 tablespoons arrowroot powder

8 drops lavender essential oil

Makes ½ cup.

Add the essential oil to the powder and mix together well. Store in a container for daily use, if desired.

To use, sprinkle all over body and rub in.

DUSTING POWDER PROMPT

Create your own skin-soothing blend of essential oils to mix into the arrowroot powder instead of lavender.

Ferreted Forest Powder

Around where I live, we have a large variety of pines, firs, and cedars. These trees are wonderful for the skin; they stimulate circulation, are full of nutrients, and nourish venous tenacity so not only do they increase circulation, but they strengthen the vein wall. They are also antimicrobial, antibacterial, and anti-fungal. I like to collect the fresh green shoots in springtime and use them in everything I possibly can.

1 cup arrowroot powder
4 tablespoons green shoots from the forest, such as pine, fir, and cedars, as available*

Makes 1 cup.

*When you're picking your shoots, make sure nothing you grab is toxic.

When you get home, mix ingredients together in a sealed jar, and shake daily. You can choose to leave the plant material in with the powder or you can strain it out. If you choose to leave it in, place powder in a jar with a shaker lid to keep plant material in when you sprinkle the powder out.

To use, sprinkle all over body and rub into skin.

PLANT POWDER PROMPT

What wild plants do you have in season around you that will safely work for skin care? Create a blend of local flora to utilize instead of the green shoots blend.

NOTES

....

....

....

....

Mists

Just like toners for the face, body mists are a good base layer before moisturizing to help tone the body all over, or just to smell amazing! Follow with a moisturizer to lock in hydration!

Basic Body Mist

1 part rose hydrosol
1 part orange blossom hydrosol

Combine the hydrosols in a bottle with a spray attachment.

To use, after bathing, shake bottle and then spritz all over body. Allow to air dry. Follow with one of the body oils in this section.

. . . .

Hydrating Frankincense and Rose Body Mist

3 ounces rose hydrosol
¼ teaspoon honey
2 drops frankincense essential oil

Makes 3 ounces.

Combine all ingredients in a bottle with a spray attachment. Shake until honey is dissolved.

To use, after bathing, shake and then spritz all over body. Allow to air dry. Follow with one of the body oils in this section. Note that this recipe has a short shelf life of about a month because of the honey, so store in refrigerator to keep from spoiling.

Forest Body Mist

3 ounces rose hydrosol

3 ounces sandalwood hydrosol

3 ounces distilled water

3 drops cypress essential oil

2 drops balsam fir absolute essential oil

2 drops pine essential oil

3 drops fir essential oil

3 drops Virginia cedarwood essential oil

2 drops thyme essential oil

2 drops rosemary essential oil

Makes 9 ounces.

Mix all ingredients together in a mason jar and shake well. Pour into containers with spritzer tops.

To use, shake mixture and spritz all over your body, avoiding contact with eyes. Air dry and follow with body oil.

Body Oils

A BIT ABOUT BODY OIL

As wonderful as extra-virgin olive oil is, it still smells like a salad, and personally, I don't prefer to smell like a salad so I don't use it on my skin. If you do like to smell like a salad, by all means, carry on with your extra-virgin olive oil slathering.

Body oils have been used extensively throughout history. During Roman times, oiling the body after a bath was a sign of status. In Ayurveda, regular oiling of the body is done for health, to pull out toxins in skin, and nourish one's very essence. It is thought that the body oil that Egyptian Queen Hatsheput used on her skin contained oils of palm, nutmeg, and a highly carcinogenic tar and quite possibly caused her demise.

I find body oil is best applied right after towel drying after bathing. At this point, your skin is moist, so when you add oil, it helps lock in moisture. Use far less oil than you expect to, as it goes further with the moisture already on your skin.

The following are my favorite recipes for body oils.

Rose and Hibiscus Oil

My favorite oils to use for body oil are jojoba and apricot kernel or plum kernel oil. These oils are non-greasy and absorb super quick while leaving your skin well nourished.

1½ ounces rose herbal oil
    (see page 22)
1½ ounces hibiscus herbal oil
    (see page 22)
1 ounce jojoba oil
1 ounce apricot kernel oil
2 drops rose essential oil or
    absolute
2 drops frankincense essential oil
4 drops bergamot essential oil

Makes 5 ounces.

Put all ingredients in jar with pump attachment and shake.

To use, shake and apply after bathing and patting dry with a towel.

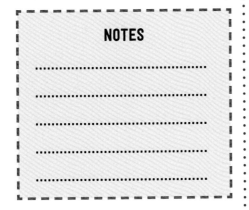

NOTES

Persephone's Blend

This fancy little oil is a blend of all-things springtime and a hint of pomegranate.

1 ounce jojoba oil
1 ounce apricot kernel oil
1 ounce sunflower oil
1 ounce argan oil
1 ounce nettle herbal oil (see page 22)
1 ounce calendula herbal oil
    (see page 22)
3 grams pomegranate oil
3 grams meadowfoam oil
4 drops bergamot essential oil
3 drops ho wood essential oil
4 drops lavender essential oil
5 drops cypress essential oil
4 drops lemon essential oil
1 drop patchouli essential oil
3 drops rosemary essential oil
4 drops grapefruit essential oil

Makes about 6½ ounces.

Put all ingredients in bottle with pump attachment and shake.

To use, shake and apply after bathing and patting dry with a towel.

Rosemary and Lavender Stimulating Body Oil

This blend enhances circulation, leading to healthy, toned skin.

1 ounce lavender and rosemary herbal oil (see page 22)
3 drops rosemary essential oil
6 drops lavender essential oil

Makes 1 ounce.

Strain lavender and rosemary herbal oil into a bottle with a pump attachment. Add essential oils. Shake well, label, and use daily.

To use, shake and apply after bathing and patting dry with a towel.

. . . .

Jasmine Body Oil

A harmonious skin melody for soft, nourished skin.

1 ounce apricot kernel oil
1 drop jasmine grandiflorum

Makes 1 ounce.

Combine ingredients in jar with a pump attachment, shake, and label.

To use, shake and apply after bathing and patting dry with a towel.

NOTES

....

....

....

....

....

BODY OIL PROMPT

Think of an attribute you would like your oil to have (calming, cooling, warming, softening, etc.).

Substitute herbal oils here with supporting herbal oils for your skin needs.

Substitute essential oils for essential oils that support your oil creation.

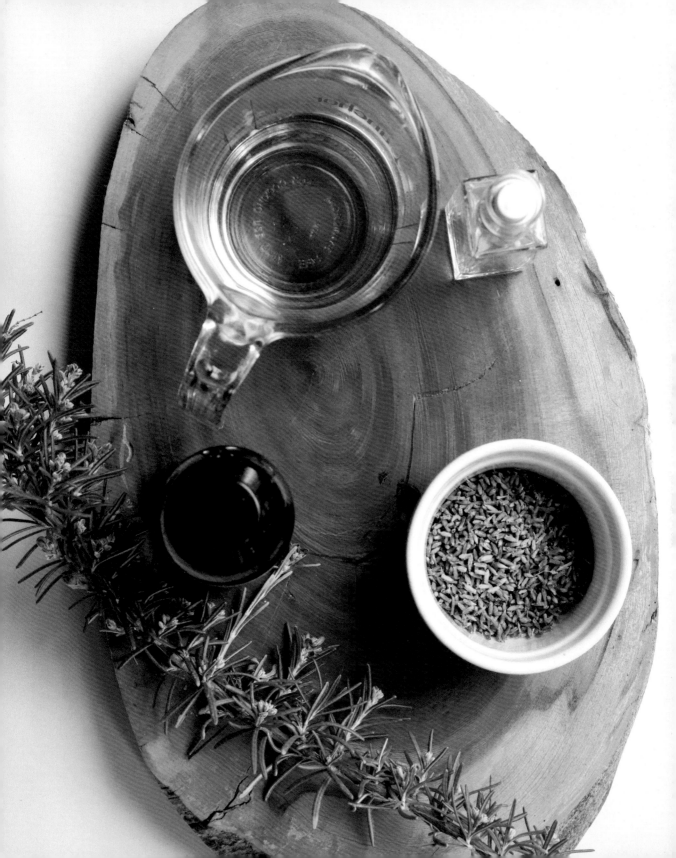

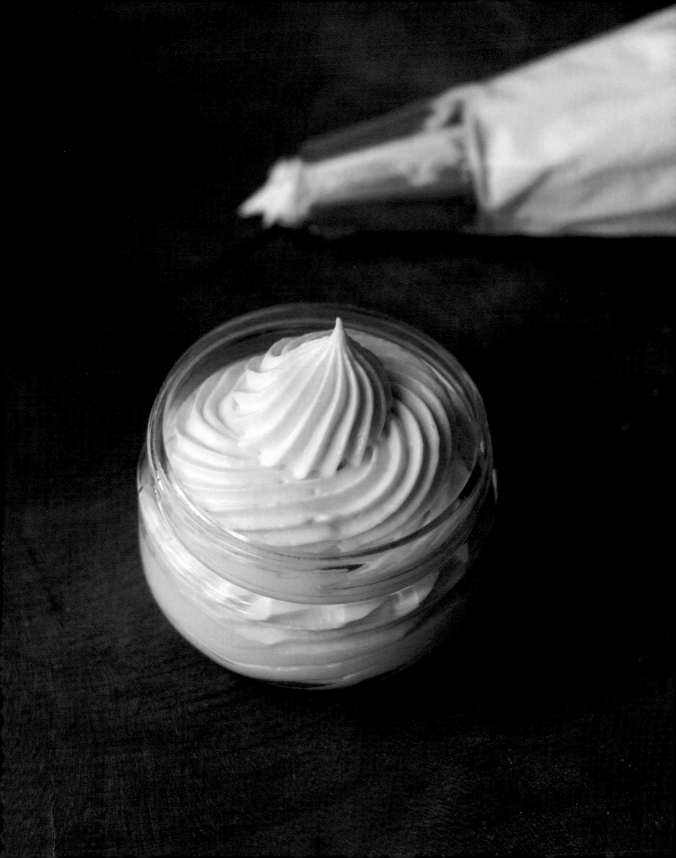

Butters

These are super rich moisturizers using heavy plant butters. They are great used in moderation, as a skin treat, and on seriously dry skin.

Whipped Body Butter

This is a delicious skin treat! Densely nourishing, wonderful for seriously dry skin or just full-body moisturizing.

2 ounces shea butter

1 ounce cocoa butter

½ ounce coconut oil

3 ounces sunflower oil

10–20 essential oils, if desired

Makes 6½ ounces.

Melt all ingredients except essential oils over a double boiler. Once melted, remove from heat and add essential oils, if using, and stir. Pour this mixture into a mixing bowl.

Set this blend in the freezer for about 5 to 10 minutes to speed solidifying. You want a malleable yet semi-solid mixture.

Using a beater, whip until creamy with soft peaks. Now you can either scoop this into containers or, for a really gorgeous look, put this whipped mixture into a frosting piping bag and pipe into containers, then cap and label.

To use, start with a pea-sized amount of butter and massage into skin. This is a super rich formula, so a little will go a long way.

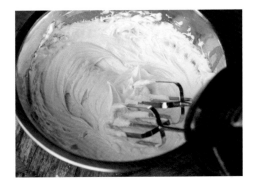

NOTES

....

....

....

....

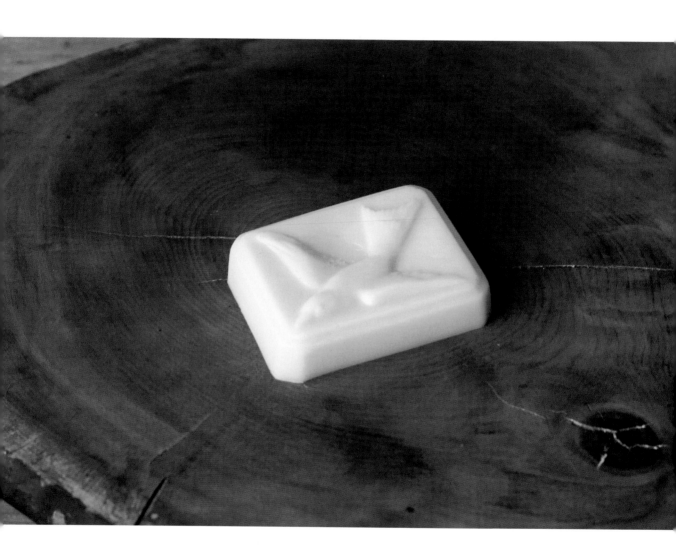

Solid Body Butter

This fun and nourishing body butter is perfect—not to mention, you can save on packaging. It's quick and easy to whip up and just a dream to apply to skin. The solid body butter gives a heavy moisturizing experience that can last all day.

20 grams beeswax
20 grams shea butter
20 grams sunflower oil

Fills one (3-ounce) mold.

Weigh out all ingredients and place in a heatproof mixing bowl. Set up a double boiler with heatproof bowl over a pan of water, turn temp to medium, and mix occasionally until melted.

Pour melted body butter into a mold. Set aside to harden, pop out of mold, and use immediately or wrap in parchment paper to use or gift later.

To use, just rub the bar all over your body and massage in.

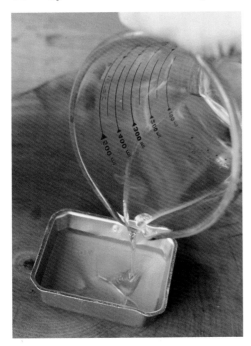

NOTES

....
....
....
....
....
....
....
....
....
....
....
....

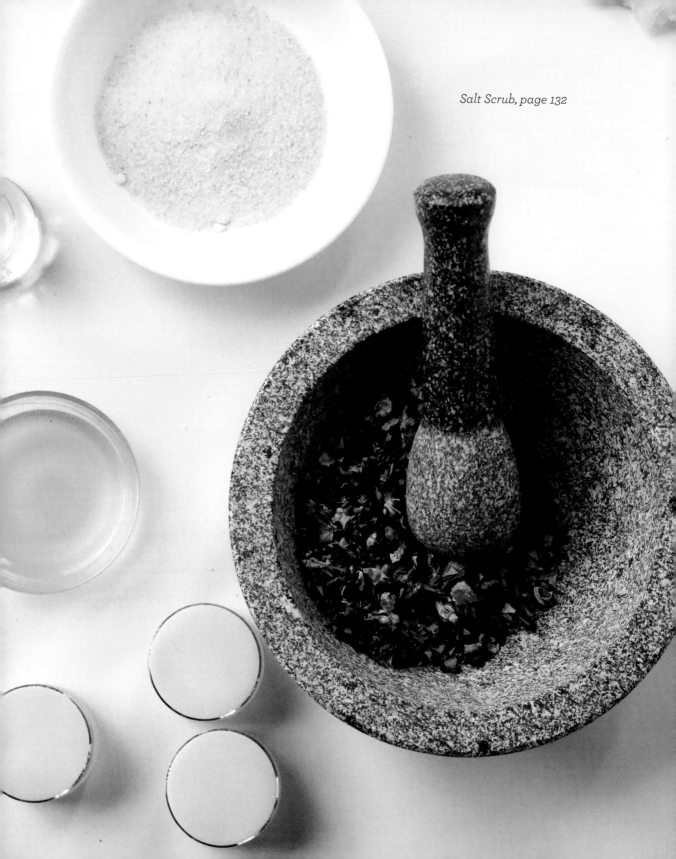

Salt Scrub, page 132

BATH

My favorite section of all! This is pure fun, functional, bath time joy. I had so much fun writing the following recipes, trying them out, and gifting them to friends. Try an exfoliating scrub, a nourishing tub tea, or a stress-reducing bath salt! Who doesn't love a good bath?

Scrubs

Scrubs are an important part of skin care as they help remove flaky dead skin and can increase healthy cellular turnover. Here's a variety to get you started.

Salt Scrub

(Body Polish)

Salt is a great pH balancer on the skin, drawing toxins, yet gently exfoliating. This recipe has just the right amount of oil and soap to get a great clean yet leave your skin soft, supple, and glowing!

1 cup salt (I used pink himalayan)

3 tablespoons dried rose petals

3 tablespoons castile soap

2 tablespoons sunflower oil

5 drops ho wood essential oil

Makes about 1¾ cups.

Mix all ingredients together well, bottle, label, and enjoy!

To use, take into shower and scrub a small amount onto wet skin. Rub in until dissolved, rinse off excess, towel dry when finished, and enjoy your incredible skin!

SALT SCRUB PROMPT

Use sugar, different salt, vary the herbs or use none at all, or try with different essential oils. This is one of those recipes that really allows you to have some fun!

NOTES

Coffee Sugar Scrub

This scrub does a lot! It exfoliates, reduces cellulite, and nourishes naturally. It's a perfect circulatory-enhancing, awesome, moisturizing sugar scrub that will leave you glowing, gently moisturized, and smooth!

120 grams organic white sugar

7 grams coffee ground or espresso

20 grams grapeseed oil (or whatever you prefer)

5 grams castile soap

1 pinch each of the following spices (optional): cinnamon, ginger, nutmeg, clove, cardamom

Makes 5½ ounces.

Blend dry ingredients together. Add wet ingredients to the dry and blend well. Scoop into jars, cap, and label.

To use, take into shower and scrub a small amount onto wet skin. Rub in until dissolved, rinse off excess, towel dry when finished, and enjoy your incredible skin!

NOTES

....

....

....

....

....

....

Coffee and warming spices stimulate circulation, aiding the body in eliminating toxin buildup that can be responsible for cellulite.

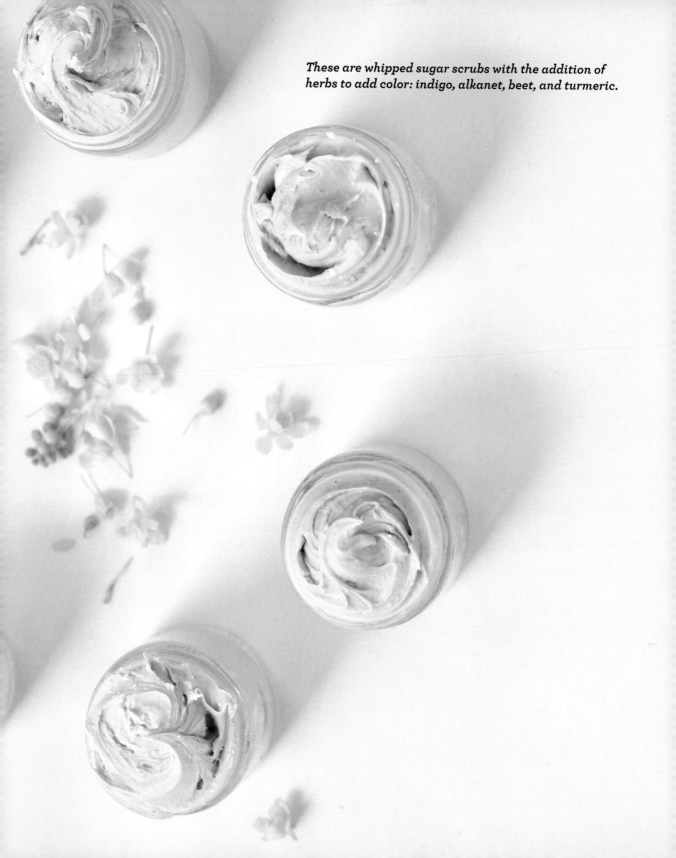

These are whipped sugar scrubs with the addition of herbs to add color: indigo, alkanet, beet, and turmeric.

Whipped Sugar Scrub

The coolest thing about this recipe is that because the arrowroot is so light and fluffy in nature, it is suspended in the cocoa butter and castile soap blend so a blender isn't necessary.

½ ounces cocoa butter
½ ounces castile soap
1 ounce castor sugar
½ ounces arrowroot powder

Makes 3½ ounces.

Simply melt cocoa butter in a heatproof container over double boiler, remove from heat when fully melted, and add in castile soap. Mix this well, and it will turn a creamy color. Add sugar and mix again before adding arrowroot. Stir until fully incorporated; it will be nice and smooth and whipped-looking. Put your mixture into containers, cap, and label.

To use this wonderful, skin softening, exfoliating, cleansing, and moisturizing blend, scoop a little into your hands and apply to wet skin. Rub in well and rinse off. Enjoy!

NOTES

I serendipitously created this recipe for you while writing this book. I was messing around in the kitchen, trying to make something else, and this came about. Part of making your own formulations will always thrive with keeping an open mind to experimentation, and as long as you learned something, there are no failures. Yes, I've tossed many, many, many more projects than I can count, but I've learned from every single one, and in the process, made some pretty cool products. This is for you.

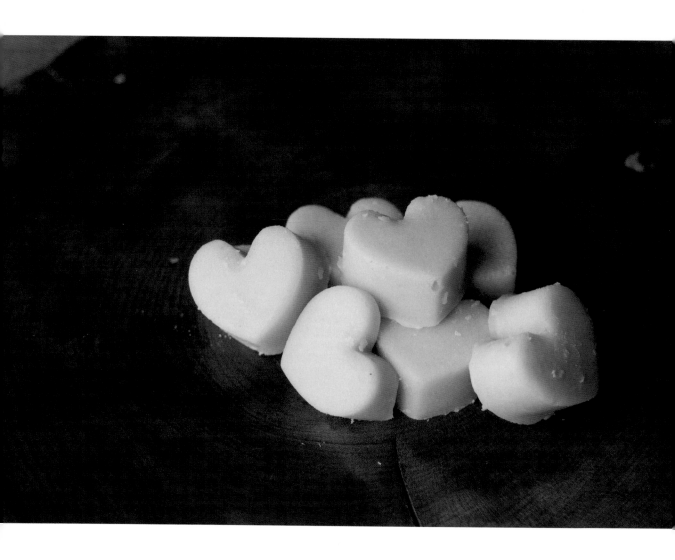

Solid Sugar Scrub

This is a super simple and straightforward recipe. Its job is to exfoliate and moisturize. I find regular sugar to be too harsh and sharp on the skin, so this recipe calls for castor sugar because it lends itself to a very lovely exfoliation.

¼ ounce coconut oil

4 ounces cocoa butter

13½ ounces castor sugar

Makes almost 18 ounces.

Melt coconut oil and cocoa butter over double boiler. When fully melted, remove from heat, add in castor sugar, and mix well.

Scoop your sugar scrub mixture into any mold you have on hand. (I like to use ice cube trays because they seem to be a perfect size.) Tap your mold on the countertop to even out the scoop of sugar scrub. Set your mold aside to solidify, or stick in the freezer for a faster solidifying time. When your scrubs are solidified, pop them out of molds, stick them in a jar, cap, and label.

To use while bathing, wet skin with warm water and gently scrub your skin all over. Rub in with more warm water until you feel fully exfoliated and marvelous. Rinse off sugar, and enjoy your well-moisturized skin!

SUGAR SCRUB PROMPT
Try adding natural powdered colors or scents to create a wide variety of sugar scrubs.

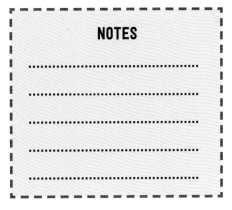

NOTES

Tub Teas and Baths

Just like tea to drink is good for your insides, a nice bath or tub tea can be great for your outsides!

Lavender and Chamomile Tub Tea

This tea is great to drink, and just as good to soak in!

1 ounce dried lavender
1 ounce dried chamomile

Makes 2 ounces of tub tea.

Put herbs into a 4x6–inch muslin bag, pull strings tight, and tie.

To use, toss bag into bathtub as it fills with warm water. Then step into bathtub and soak!

Feel free to omit the bag if you don't mind floating herbs in your bath. In that case, simply put herbs in a jar instead and scoop into bath with a spoon.

. . . .

Milk Bath

Milk is incredibly soothing and softening for the skin. You can use any type of dried milk powder you like.

1 cup powdered coconut milk
1 tablespoon shaved cocoa butter bits
2 tablespoons hibiscus

Makes about 1 cup of milk bath.

Place all ingredients in a bowl and mix well. Pour mixture into jar with lid, cap, label.

To use, pour ingredients into bathtub and fill bath with warm water. Step into tub and soak!

Soothing Oatmeal Bath

This is a wonderful blend for dry skin, irritated skin, flaky patches, and poison oak.

1 cup oats, ground to powder
1 tablespoon powdered nettle
1 tablespoon powdered astragalus
1 tablespoon powdered lemon balm

Makes about 1 cup of oatmeal bath.

Mix all ingredients together, bottle, cap, and label.

To use, scoop three tablespoons into running bath water, soak, and enjoy!

. . . .

Chocolate and Roses Bath

1 cup magnesium salt (Epsom salt)
1 teaspoon honey
1 teaspoon cocoa butter shavings
1 tablespoon rose petals
1½ tablespoons cocoa powder
⅛ teaspoon vanilla powder

Makes about 1¼ cups.

Measure out the magnesium salt and add the honey. Squish honey into salt with your hands until well incorporated, then add the rest of the ingredients. Stir (or squish!) to combine. Pour into jar, cap, and label.

To use, pour any amount you'd like (as little as 2 tablespoons and as much as the whole mixture) into running bath water and mix in. Bathe, enjoy!

Bath Salts

A NOTE ABOUT BASIC BATH SALTS

I use magnesium sulfate (Epsom salt) for almost all my bath salts and add just a bit of other salts if I want variety. Magnesium has incredible stress-reducing abilities; our bodies cannot digest basic life stressors without it.

This is why you soak injured body parts in magnesium baths; it brings down swelling and inflammation, it increases healing, and it decreases pain and bruising because it literally helps your body take care of that physical stress. If you have shaky or painful hands from arthritis, magnesium soaks can help. If you want to increase healing of broken bones—magnesium. If you are having anxiety, emotional upsets, shock from trauma, or are grieving, use magnesium. It helps our bodies digest emotional stress, too!

Just make sure to use on closed skin only.

Another fun fact about magnesium is that, as important as it is for us, we have a hard time digesting it. It goes straight through our bodies, which is why, internally, it works so well as a laxative. However, we can absorb it very well through our skin (transdermal absorption). No need to worry about absorbing too much this way because our bodies are magical and don't allow that to occur, which is why super-saturated flotation tank therapy works so well.

I could go on and on about magnesium, but I think you get the gist.

Other salts are great, but they just aren't magnesium. That being said, other salts have varying mineral contents, so I like to add certain ones, for skin health, to Epsom salt blends.

Basic Bath Salts

2 cups Epsom salt

2 ounces essential oil of your choice

2 tablespoons dried herbs of your choice

Makes about 2 cups of bath salts.

Mix all ingredients together, bottle, cap, and label.

To use, pour a few tablespoons or half the batch into warm running bath water. Immerse your body, soak, and enjoy!

Elder and Orange Bath Salts

Orange and elder is a soothing, uplifting blend, helping to invoke feelings of joy.

2 cups Epsom salt
4 drops patchouli essential oil
10 drops bergamot essential oil
10 drops sweet orange essential oil
10 drops blood orange essential oil
1 tablespoon dried elder flowers
1 tablespoon dried orange peel bits

Makes about 2 cups.

Mix Epsom salts and essential oils well, add herbs, and mix again. Scoop into jar and label.

To use, pour 2 tablespoons or up to the whole jar into the bathtub and run warm bath water. Step into bath, soak, and enjoy.

NOTES

....
....
....
....
....
....
....

Fizzing Bath Salts

These add an effervescent twist to bath time with their instant fizz when they hit the water. My kids love these!

½ cup baking soda
2 cups Epsom salt
essential oils if desired
¼ cup citric acid
⅛ cup arrowroot powder

Makes about 3 cups.

Mix Epsom salts and essential oils well, add powders, mix, scoop into jar, label.

To use, pour 2 tablespoons or up to the whole jar into the bath, run warm bath water, step into bath, enjoy.

NOTES

....
....
....
....
....
....
....

Extras

Just for fun, theses are wonderful additives to invoke a joyous bathing experience for all ages.

Whole Body Green Tea Skin Mask

Revitalize skin with invigorating antioxidant-rich green tea while pulling out toxins and toning skin with this delightful recipe!

3 ounces Basic Facial Mask (see page 56)

6 ounces glycerin

1 ounce green tea powder (matcha)

1 ounce arrowroot powder

Makes 11 ounces.

Blend all ingredients together in a bottle, cap, and label.

To use, apply a small amount to wet skin, rub in, rinse off, and enjoy your refreshed skin!

. . . .

Basic Bath Bomb

Bath bombs are an easily varied recipe, great to try out with various herbs colors, scents, and shapes.

2–3 tablespoons coconut oil

1 cup baking soda

½ cup citric acid

¼ cup arrowroot powder

essential oils, if desired

1–3 teaspoons distilled water or hydrosol in spritzer bottle

Makes about 2 cups.

Melt coconut oil over double boiler. While coconut oil is melting, blend together powder ingredients in a mixing bowl. Once coconut oil is melted, slowly pour half of it over your powder mixtures and blend. Mixing with your hands to

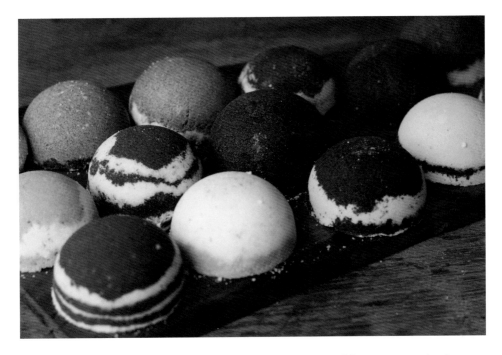

crush lumps, then add the rest of the oil. If you are adding essential oils, now is the time.

Spray about 8 spritzes with your water over the mixture and keep moving with your hands until mixture just starts holding together. Once mixture is holding together, press some firmly into a mold design of your choice. Fill mold and press as hard as you can to create a solid cake.

Now, line a cookie sheet with freezer paper and hit your mold against the cookie sheet so the bath bomb pops out. Leave on cookie sheet for 24 hours in a safe, dry place. Then, wrap in parchment or waxed paper and label.

To use, pop in a warm bath and watch the magic happen!

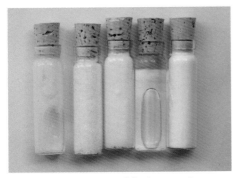

coconut oil, citric acid, baking soda, distilled water, arrowroot powder

BATH BOMB PROMPT

What types of ground herbs could you add to create colorful bath bombs?

143

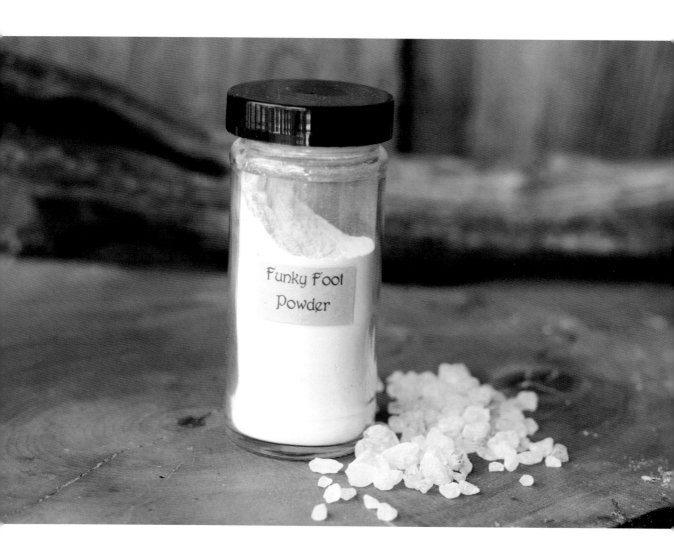

FEET

I love caring for feet. They are our foundation and they take us anywhere we want to go. They deserve a lot of love and care. For an excellent foot pampering session, start with the exfoliating Foot Scrub (page 146), follow with either the Soothing Foot Soak (page 147), or Foot Fizzies (page 148). Dry your feet off and finish with a Funky Foot Powder (page 149) for the happiest, sweetest scented feet ever!

Foot Scrub

This stimulating exfoliating and softening blend is a great way to start pampering your feet. Just be careful because it may cause your step to be extra slippery.

½ cup salt (I used pink Himalayan).

½ cup sugar

½ cup baking soda

3 tablespoons castile soap

2 tablespoons sunflower oil

5 drops eucalyptus essential oil

2 drops lemongrass essential oil

5 drops rosemary essential oil

Makes about 1 cup of scrub.

Mix all ingredients together well, scoop into a jar, cap, label, enjoy!

To use, either in bath or in a foot soak, wet feet, scoop a little scrub into hands, and massage into one foot at a time.

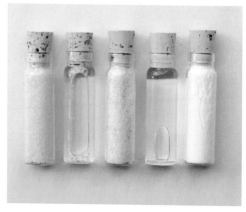

organic sugar, castile soap, pink himalayan salt, sunflower oil, baking soda

Soothing Foot Soak

This is a really simple blend, but those magnesium salts mixed with stimulating deodorizing eucalyptus makes for a potent formula of relaxation and enhanced circulation. Take the edge off foot pain, balance pH levels so your feet don't stink, soothe sore feet with stimulating eucalyptus.

1 cup Epsom salt
5 drops eucalyptus essential oil*

Makes 1 cup of soak.

Add essential oil to cup of Epsom salt, mix, and pour into a jar. Cap, label, and enjoy!

To use, scoop anywhere between 2 tablespoons and the whole cup into a tub or foot bath of warm water, soak feet, and relax!

*Feel free to use dried eucalyptus as well or instead of essential oil.

FOOT SOAK PROMPT

What other essential oils or blends would be exceptionally wonderful for feet? Consider the condition of your feet. Which would be perfect for them?

NOTES

....

....

....

....

....

....

Groovy Foot Fizzies

Try sprinkling flower petals or colorants in the bottom of your tray before pressing in the foot fizzie mixture.

2–3 tablespoons coconut oil

1 cup baking soda

½ cup citric acid

¼ cup arrowroot powder

½ cup magnesium sulfate

3 drops patchouli essential oil

4 drops lemon essential oil

2 drops ginger essential oil

1 drop cardamom essential oil

2 drops nutmeg essential oil

10 drops sweet orange essential oil

1–2 teaspoons distilled water in spritzer bottle

Makes about 2½ cups.

Melt coconut oil over double boiler. While coconut oil is melting, blend together powder ingredients in a mixing bowl. Once coconut oil is melted, slowly pour half of it over your powder mixture and blend. You'll probably have to mix with your hands to crush lumps. Add the rest of the oil and then essential oils. Now spritz about 8 sprays of your water over mixture and keep working with your hands until mixture just starts holding together.

Once mixture is holding together, press it firmly into a mold of your choice. Fill up mold by pressing as hard as you can. Let sit for about 15 to 30 minutes.

Line a cookie sheet with freezer paper and hit your mold against the cookie sheet so the foot fizzies pop out. Leave on cookie sheet for 24 hours, and then wrap in parchment or waxed paper and label.

To use, pop in a warm foot bath and watch the magic happen. Immerse your feet and feel the joy!

NOTES

....

....

....

Funky Foot Powder

(Foot Deodorant Powder)
Keep foot funk under control with this moisture-absorbing powder that reduces bacterial growth and keeps your feet smelling sweet all day long!

¼ cup arrowroot powder

1 cup bentonite clay

⅓ cup kaolin clay

½ tablespoon frankincense powder

½ tablespoon myrrh powder

10 drops lavender essential oil

Makes about 2 cups of dust.

Mix all ingredients together, place in container with a shaker lid, label, and enjoy.

To use, apply to feet before putting on shoes and as needed. This blend may make your feet slippery on hard flooring so use caution.

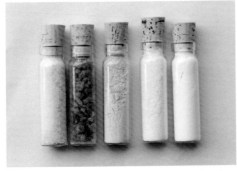

frankincense, myrrh, bentonite clay, kaolin clay, arrowroot powder

NOTES

149

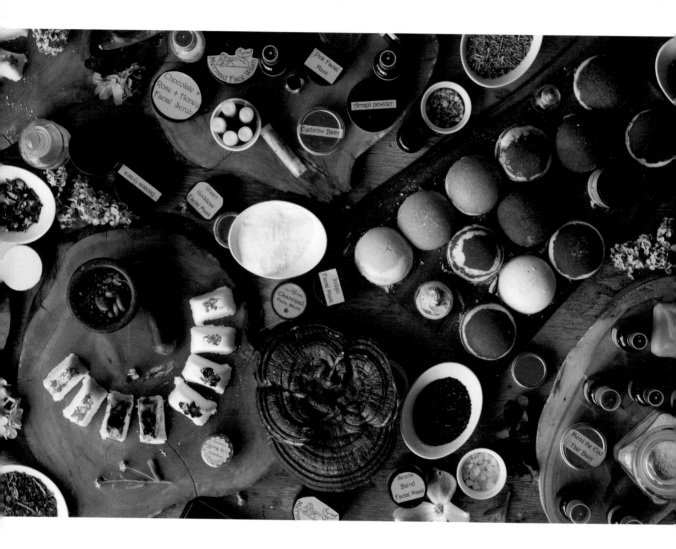

Gift Set Ideas

Get creative with wrapping and labeling, use fun jars—you can keep it simple or get as fancy as you like. For labeling, I like to type a label up on the computer and print it to a sheet of sticker paper, which I cut to size and apply. If you have great penmanship, there's nothing as lovely as a handwritten label.

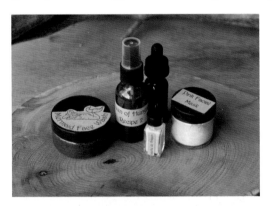

Facial Bliss

Pink Facial Mask (page 61)

Mermaid Face Wash (page 49)

Queen of Hungary's Waters (page 70)

Leche de Dragon blemish reducer (page 80)

Your choice of moisturizer (pages 83–86)

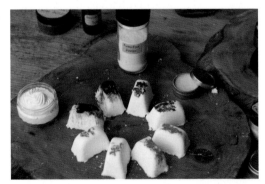

Foot Love

Groovy Foot Fizzies (page 148)

Funky Foot Powder (page 149)

Cuticle Cream (page 112)

Whipped Body Butter (page 127)

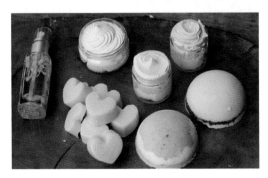

Bath Lover

Basic Bath Bomb (page 142)

Solid Sugar Scrub (page 137)

Whipped Sugar Scrub (page 135)

Whipped Body Butter (page 127)

Jasmine Body Oil (page 124)

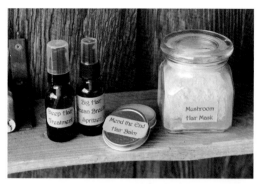

Basic Hair Care

Deep Hair Treatment (page 31)

Big Hair Ocean Breeze Spritzer
(page 33)

Mend the End Hair Balm
(page 35)

Mushroom Hair Mask (page 37)

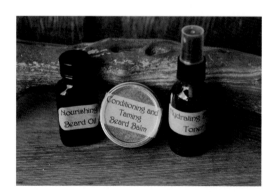

Serious Hair Care

Deep Hair Treatment (page 31)

Big Hair Ocean Breeze Spritzer
(page 33)

Mend the End Hair Balm (page 35)

Mushroom Hair Mask (page 37)

Perfumed Hair Mist (page 33)

Stimulating Scalp Oil (page 29)

Healthy Shiny Hair Oil (page 26)

Beard Love

Hydrating Beard Toner (page 43)

Nourishing Beard Oil (page 39)

Beard Conditioning Taming
Balm (page 41)

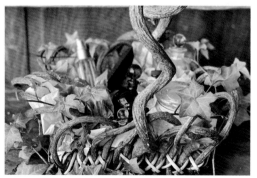

Head to Toe

One of everything you've made from each section! I do this regularly for gifting. I'll take one of everything I have available and wrap them all up. People LOVE it!

Resources

Feel free to contact the me if you have questions about the ingredients or materials used in this book. You can reach me by visiting my business's website: MoonMagic.co. I love to hear from my readers!

ESSENTIAL OILS

Floracopeia | www.floracopeia.com
13100 Grass Valley Ave., Suite D
Grass Valley CA 95945
Phone: 866-417-1149

Eden Botanicals | www.edenbotanicals.com
3820 Cypress Dr. #12
Petaluma, CA 94954
Phone: 707-509-0041

The Perfumery | www.theperfumery.com
621 Park East Blvd
New Albany, IN 47150
Phone: 502-498-8804

White Lotus Aromatics | www.whitelotusaromatics.com
941 E. Snowline Dr.
Port Angeles, WA 98362
Phone: 360-683-0137

The Herbarie | www.theherbarie.com
The Herbarie at Stoney Hill Farm, Inc.
630 Turner Rd
Prosperity, SC 29127
Phone: 803-364-9979

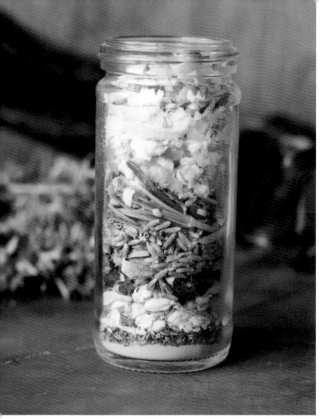

Queen of Hungary's Water II, page 70

Starwest Botanicals | www.starwest-botanicals.com
161 Main Ave
Sacramento, CA 95838
Toll-free: (800) 800-4372

ESSENTIAL OILS, BULK OILS, CLAYS, HERBS

Prima Fluer | www.primafleur.com
84 Galli Drive
Novato, CA 94949
Phone: 415-455-0957

Mountain Rose Herbs | www.mountainroseherbs.com
PO Box 50220
Eugene, OR 97405
Phone: 800-879-3337

Liberty Natural Products | www.libertynatural.com
The Oregon Lavender Farm
20949 S. Harris Road
Oregon City, OR 97045
Phone: 800-289-8427

Camden-Grey Essential Oils | www.camdengrey.com
5751 Halifax Ave. #2
Fort Myers, FL 33912
Phone: 305-500-9630

Monterey Bay Spice Company | www.herbco.com
241 Walker Street
Watsonville, CA 95076
Phone: 800-500-6148

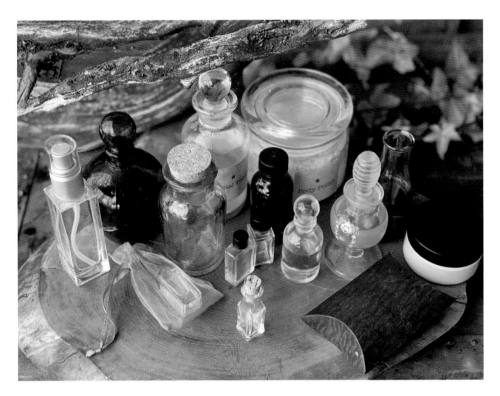

Essential Depot | www.essentialdepot.com
2029 US Hwy 27 South,
Sebring, FL 33875
Phone: 866-840-2495

Bramble Berry Soap Making Supplies | www.brambleberry.com
2138 Humboldt St.
Bellingham, WA 98225
Phone: 360-734-8278

Bulk Apothecary | www.bulkapothecary.com
125 Lena Drive
Aurora, Ohio 44202
Phone: 888-728-7612

BOTTLES

Glass Bottle Outlet | www.glassbottleoutlet.com
110 West Interlake Boulevard
Lake Placid FL 33852
Phone: 888-395-6551 or 863-655-2210

Nemat International | www.nematinternational.com
34135 7th Street
Union City, CA 94587
Phone: 1-800-936-3628

Berlin Packaging | www.berlinpackaging.com
525 West Monroe Street
Chicago, IL 60661
Phone: 800-7-BERLIN (800-723-7546)

ALCOHOL FOR TINCTURES

The Organic Alcohol Company | www.organicalcohol.com
650 Mistletoe Road
Ashland, Oregon 97520
Phone: 866-801-1050

GENERAL

Etsy is a great place to find a variety of supplies, as well as a good place to start selling your own products, should you so wish to do so.
www.etsy.com

Index